Definitive Anti Inflammatory Diet Cookbook

Delicious and on a Budget Dessert Recipes to Boost your Metabolism

Zac Gibson

Table of Contents

Strawberry Ice Cream

Prep Time:
5 minutes
Cook Time:
5 minutes
Serve: 2-3

Ingredients:

- 1 Banana, frozen & cut
- 1 cup Strawberries, frozen
- 1 tsp. Vanilla extract
- 2 tbsp. Coconut Milk

Directions:

1.Begin by placing strawberries and banana in a high-speed blender and blend it for two to three minutes.

2.While you blend, spoon in the coconut milk, and the vanilla extract.

3.Carry on blending until the mixture is thick and smooth.

4.Serve the ice-cream instantly since it does not keep well in the freezer.

Nutrition: ‖ Calories: 78 Kcal ‖ Protein: 1g ‖ Carbohydrates: 13.6g ‖ Fat:2.7g

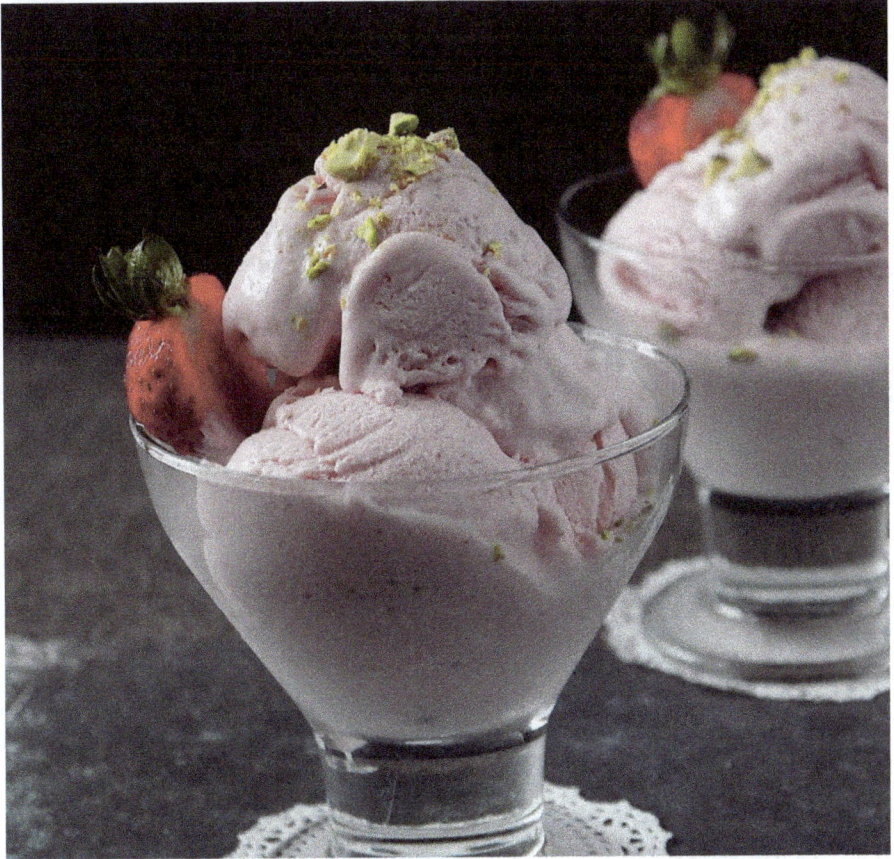

Strawberry Orange Sorbet

Prep Time:
5 minutes
Cook Time:
0 minutes
Serve: 3

Ingredients:

- 1 cup Orange juice or coconut water
- 1 pound Frozen strawberries

Directions:

1.Pour strawberries in a blender and pulse until all you have left are flakes. two minutes tops.

2.Now put in the coconut water or orange juice and pulse until you get a nice and smooth puree.

3.Have a spatula handy because you might need to scrape some of the puree off the walls of the blender sometimes.

4.Serve the moment you're done or put in the freezer for about forty- five minutes for a sorbet feel.

5.Also, you can pour the smoothie into popsicle molds and freeze for hours or even overnight.

Nutrition: ‖ Calories: 118 kcal ‖ Protein: 2.88 g ‖ Fat: 2.19 g ‖ Carbohydrates: 23.25 g

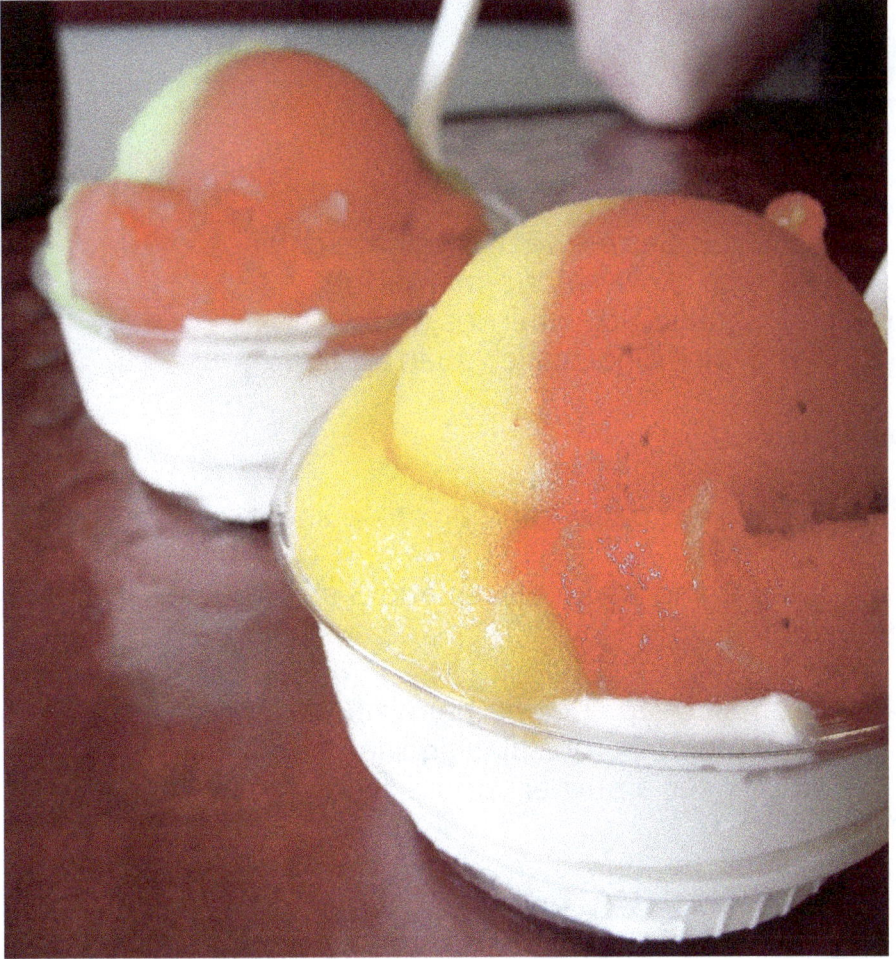

Strawberry Shortcake

Prep Time:
15 minutes
Cook Time:
0 minutes
 Serve: 4

Ingredients:

- 25 cup Semi-sweet chocolate chips
- 1 tbsp. Low-calorie margarine
- 12 hulled Strawberries
- 2.3-inch Shortcake, quartered

Directions:

1.Using waxed paper, line a cookie sheet.

2.Thread 2 shortcake pieces and 3 strawberries on 4 skewers.

3.In a small deep cooking pan, mix the margarine and chocolate chips before placing the deep cooking pan on the stove over a burner turned to low heat.

4.Stir until the ingredients are well mixed.

5.Sprinkle the chocolate onto the kabobs and then put them in your fridge for about four minutes to cool.

Nutrition: ‖ Calories: 40 kcal ‖ Protein: 1.85 g ‖ Fat: 2.3 g ‖
Carbohydrates: 3.32 g

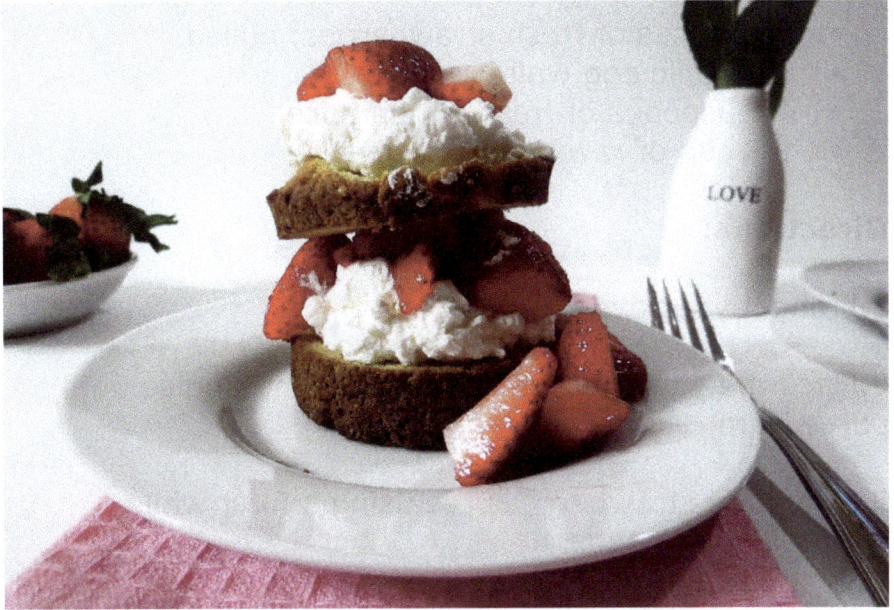

Strawberry Soufflé

Prep Time:
15 minutes
Cook Time:
20 minutes
Serve: 6

Ingredients:

- 18 ounces of fresh strawberries, hulled
- 5 organic egg whites, divided
- 4 teaspoons of fresh lemon juice
- 1/3 cup of raw honey, divided

Directions:

1.Preheat your oven to 350F.

2.Place the strawberries in a blender then pulse until a puree form.

3.Strain the strawberry puree using a filter while discarding the seeds.

4.Mix the strawberry puree to three tablespoons of honey, two egg whites, and fresh lemon juice. Pulse until a frothy and light-weight develops.

5.Beat the eggs in a separate container up to it becomes frothy.

6.Put in the remaining honey and beat until a stiff peak forms.

7.Gently- fold the egg whites into the strawberry mixture.

8.Move the mixture toto six big ramekins and place them on a baking sheet.

9.Bake for around 10-twelve minutes.

10.Take out of the oven and serve instantly.

Nutrition: ‖ Calories: 100 ‖ Fat: 0.3g ‖ Carbohydrates: 22.3g ‖ Sugar: 19.9g ‖ Protein: 3.7g ‖ Sodium: 30mg

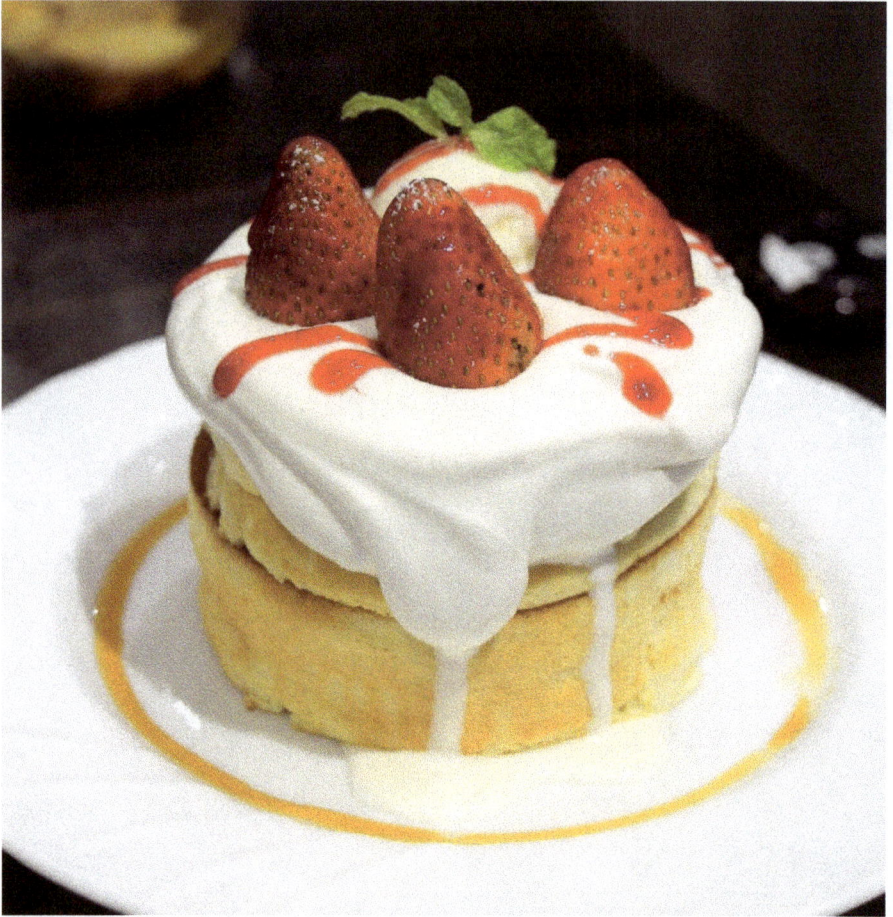

Sweet Almond And Coconut Fat Bombs

Prep Time:
10 minutes + 20 minutes chill time
Cook Time:
0 minutes
Serve: 4

Ingredients:

- ¼ cup melted coconut oil
- 3 tablespoons cocoa
- 9 and ½ tablespoons almond butter
- 9 tablespoons melted almond butter, sunflower seeds
- 90 drops liquid stevia

Directions:

1.Take a container and put in all of the listed ingredients

2.Combine them well

3.Pour scant 2 tablespoons of the mixture into as many muffin molds as you prefer

4.Chill for about twenty minutes and pop them out

Nutrition: ‖ Total Carbohydrates: 2g ‖ Fiber: 0g ‖ Protein: 2.53g ‖ Fat: 14g

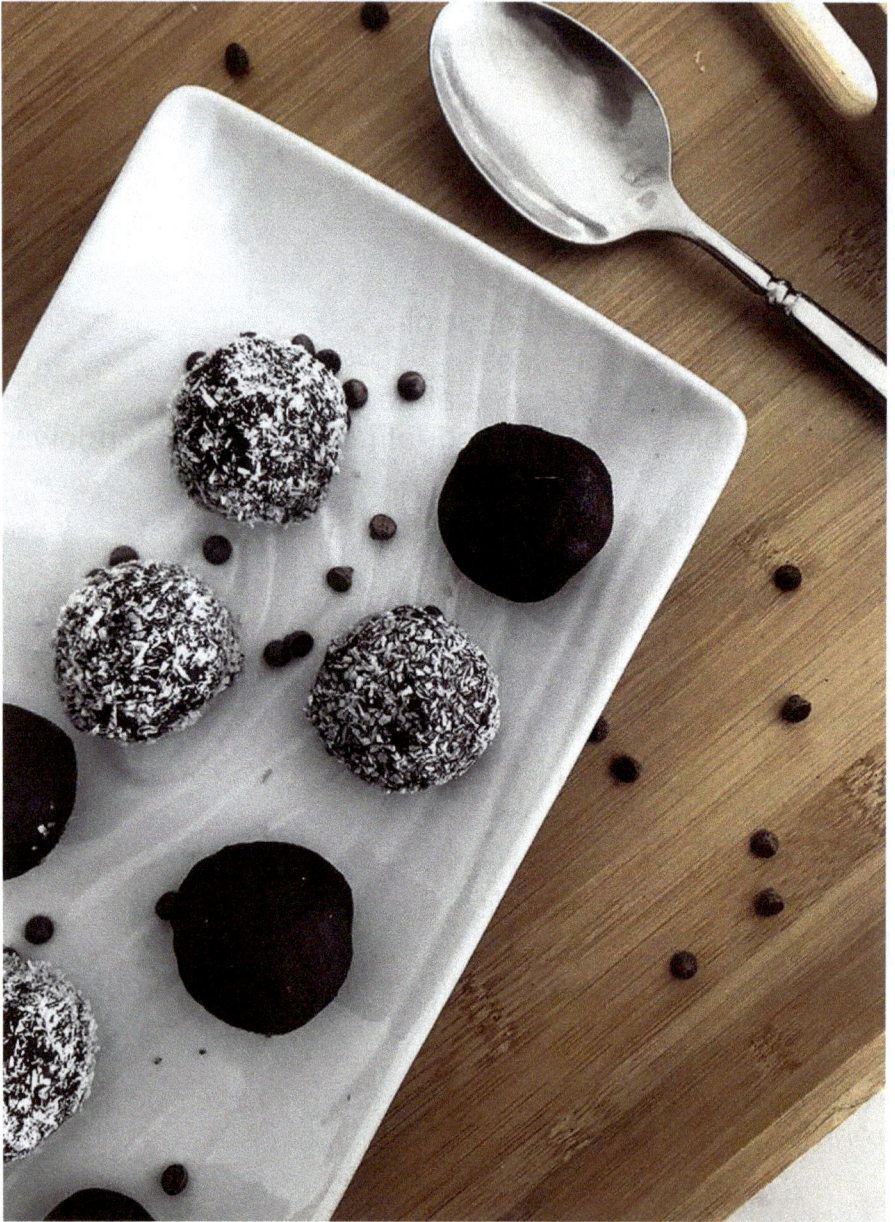

The Most Elegant Parsley Soufflé Ever

Prep Time:
5 minutes
Cook Time:
6 minutes
Serve: 5

Ingredients:

- 1 fresh red chili pepper, chopped
- 1 tablespoon fresh parsley, chopped
- 2 tablespoons coconut cream
- 2 whole eggs Sunflower seeds to taste

Directions:

1.Preheat the oven to 390 degrees F

2.Almond butter 2 soufflé dishes

3.Place the ingredients to a blender and mix thoroughly

4.Split batter into soufflé dishes and bake for about six minutes

Nutrition: ‖ Calories: 108 ‖ Fat: 9g ‖ Carbohydrates: 9g ‖ Protein: 6g

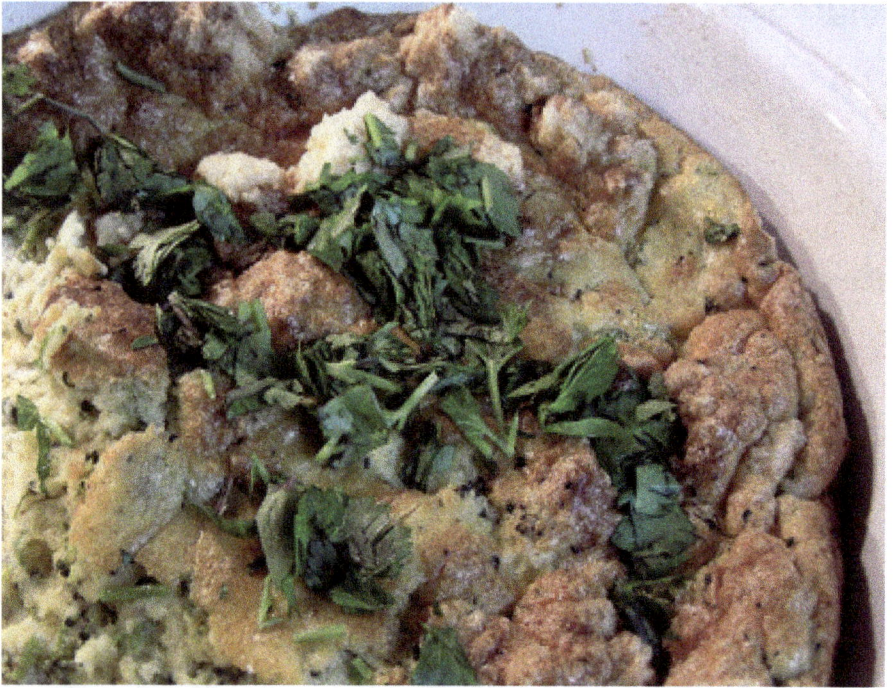

Tropical Fruit Crisp

Prep Time:
10 minutes
Cook Time:
15 minutes
Serve: 6

Ingredients:

For the Filling:

- 1 big mango (cut into chunks)
- 1 big pineapple (cut into chunks)
- 1/8 teaspoon of ground cinnamon
- 1/8 teaspoon of ground ginger
- 2 tablespoons of coconut oil
- 2 tablespoons of coconut sugar

For the Topping:

- ¾ cup of almonds
- ½ teaspoon of ground allspice
- ½ teaspoon of ground cinnamon
- ½ teaspoon of ground ginger
- 1/3 cup of unsweetened coconut, shredded

Directions:

1.Preheat your oven to 375 degrees F.

2.To make the filling: melt the coconut oil in a pan on medium-low heat and cook the coconut sugar for a couple of minutes while stirring.

3.Put in the rest of the ingredients then cook for minimum five minutes. Stir.

4.Take away the contents from heat and move it to a baking dish.

5.For the topping: Combine all ingredients in a mixer and pulse until a coarse meal forms.

6.Put the topping over the filling.

7.Bake for minimum fifteen minutes or until the top becomes golden brown.

Nutrition: ‖ Calories: 265 ‖ Fat: 12.4g ‖ Carbohydrates: 38g ‖ Sugar: 23.3g ‖ Protein: 4.3g ‖ Sodium: 17mg

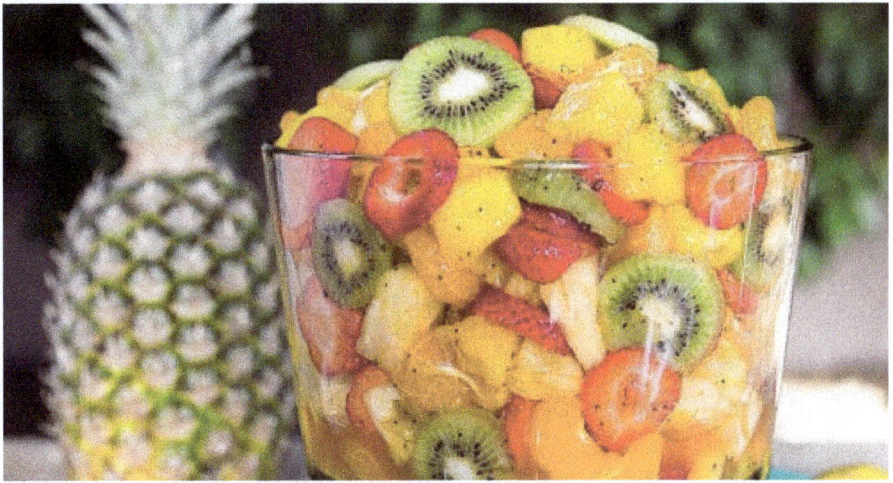

Tropical Popsicles

Prep Time:
10 minutes
Cook Time:
10 minutes
 Serve: 6

Ingredients:

- ½ tsp. Black Pepper
- 2 Kiwi, cut
- 2 tbsp. Coconut Oil
- 2 tsp. Turmeric
- 3 cups Pineapple, chopped

Directions:

1.First, place all the ingredients needed to make the popsicles excluding the kiwi in a high-speed blender for a couple of minutes or until you get a smooth mixture.

2.After this, pour the smoothie into the popsicle molds.

3.Next, insert the kiwi slices into the molds and then put the frames in the freezer until set.

4.Tip: If you desire texture, you can blend it less.

Nutrition: ‖ Calories: 101 Kcal ‖ Protein: 0.5g ‖ Carbohydrates: 15g ‖ Fat:4g

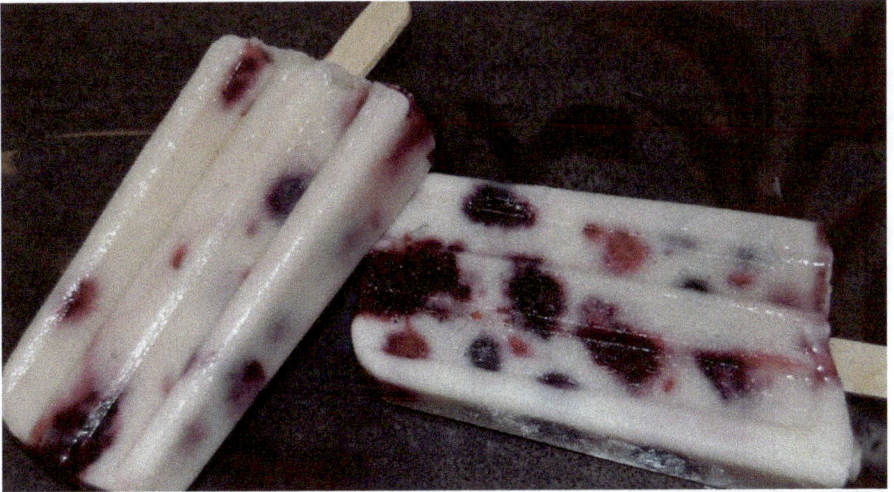

Turmeric Milkshake

Prep Time:
5 minutes
Cook Time:
0 minutes
Serve: 2

Ingredients:

- 1 tablespoon of ground flaxseeds
- 1 teaspoon of turmeric
- 2 cups of unsweetened almond milk
- 2 frozen bananas
- 2 tablespoons of raw cocoa powder
- 3 tablespoons of raw honey

Directions:

1.Combine all ingredients into a high-speed blender, and blend until the desired smoothness is achieved.

2.Split between two serving glasses, and enjoy straight away.

Nutrition: ‖ Total Carbohydrates: 74g ‖ Fiber: 7g ‖ Protein: 4g ‖ Total Fat: 6g ‖ Calories: 334

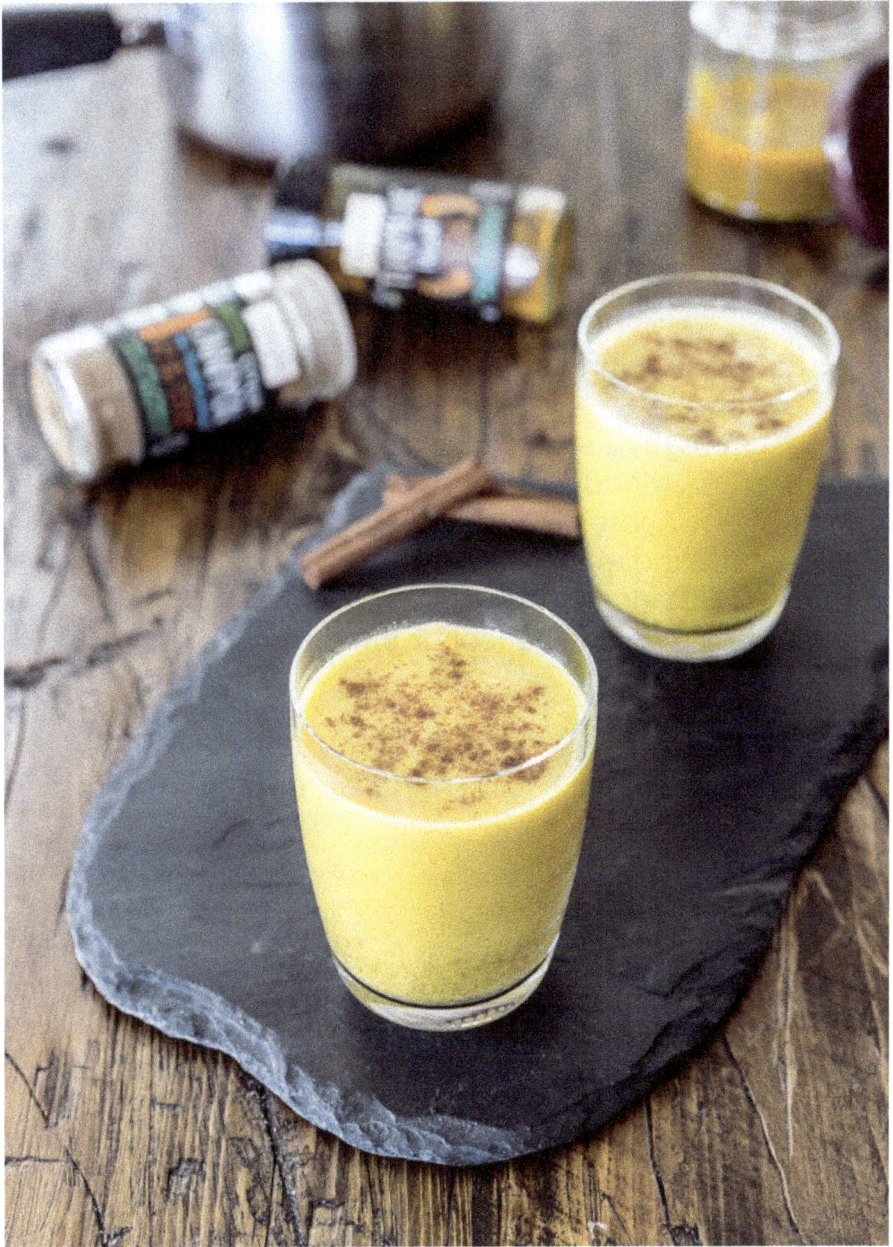

Vanilla Cakes

Prep Time:
10 minutes
Cook Time:
15 minutes
Serve: 8

Ingredients:

- .5 tsp. Baking soda
- .5 tsp. Salt
- 1 cup Agave sweetener
- 1 cup Almond milk
- 1 tbsp. Apple cider vinegar
- 2 cup Whole wheat flour
- 2 tsp. Baking powder
- C.5 cup warmed coconut oil tsp.
- Vanilla extract

Directions:

1.Ensure the oven is set to 350F.

2.Prepare two muffin pans (12 c) for use by greasing them.

3.Put in the apple cider vinegar into a measuring c that is big enough to hold minimum 2 c.

4.Put in in the almond milk for a total of 1.5 c. Allow the results to curdle roughly five minutes or until done.

5.Put together the salt, baking soda, baking powder, sugar, and flour together in a big container and whisk well.

6.Separately, mix the vanilla, coconut oil, and curdled almond in its container before combining the two bowls and blending well. Put in the results to the muffin pans, dividing uniformly.

7.Put the muffin pans in your oven and allow them to cook for approximately fifteen minutes. You will know if it's all already cook when you can press down on the tops and spring back when pressed lightly.

8.Allow the cake pans to cool on a wire rack before removing the cakes for the best results.

Nutrition: ‖ Calories: 336 kcal ‖ Protein: 5.75 g ‖ Fat: 16.25 g ‖ Carbohydrates: 44.15 g

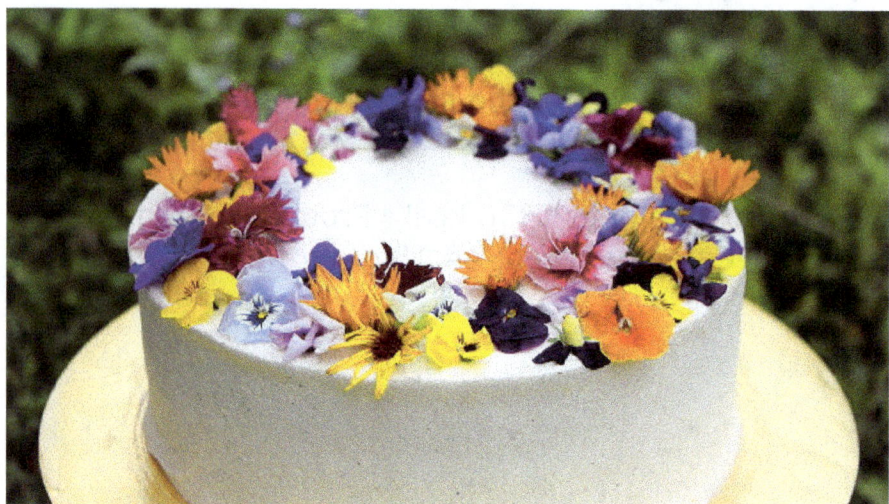

Watermelon And Avocado Cream

Prep Time:
2 hours
Cook Time:
0 minutes
Serve: 4

Ingredients:

- 1 tablespoon honey
- 1 watermelon, peeled and chopped
- 2 avocados, peeled, pitted and chopped
- 2 cups coconut cream
- 2 teaspoons lemon juice

Directions:

1.Throw all the ingredients into a blender.

2.Split it into bowls, and keep in your refrigerator for about two hours before you serve.

Nutrition: Calories 121 ‖ Fat: 2 ‖ Fiber: 2 ‖ Carbohydrates: 6 ‖ Protein: 5

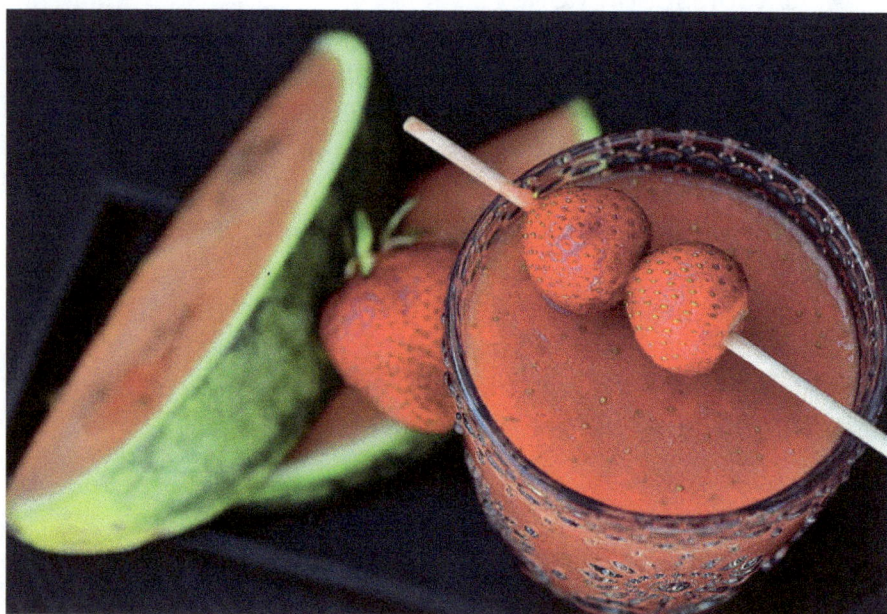

Watermelon Sorbet

Prep Time:
5 minutes
Cook Time:
15 minutes
Serve: 4

Ingredients:

- 1 Seedless Watermelon, cubed

Directions:

1.To start with, put the watermelon cubes in a baking sheet in a uniform layer.

2.Next, keep the sheet in the freezer for about two hours or until the watermelon is solid.

3.After this, move the frozen watermelon cubes in the high-speed blender and puree them until you get a smooth puree.

4.Next, pour the puree among the two loaf pans.

Nutrition: ‖ Calories: 427Kcal ‖ Protein:5.9g ‖ Carbohydrates: 80g ‖ Fat: 15.6g

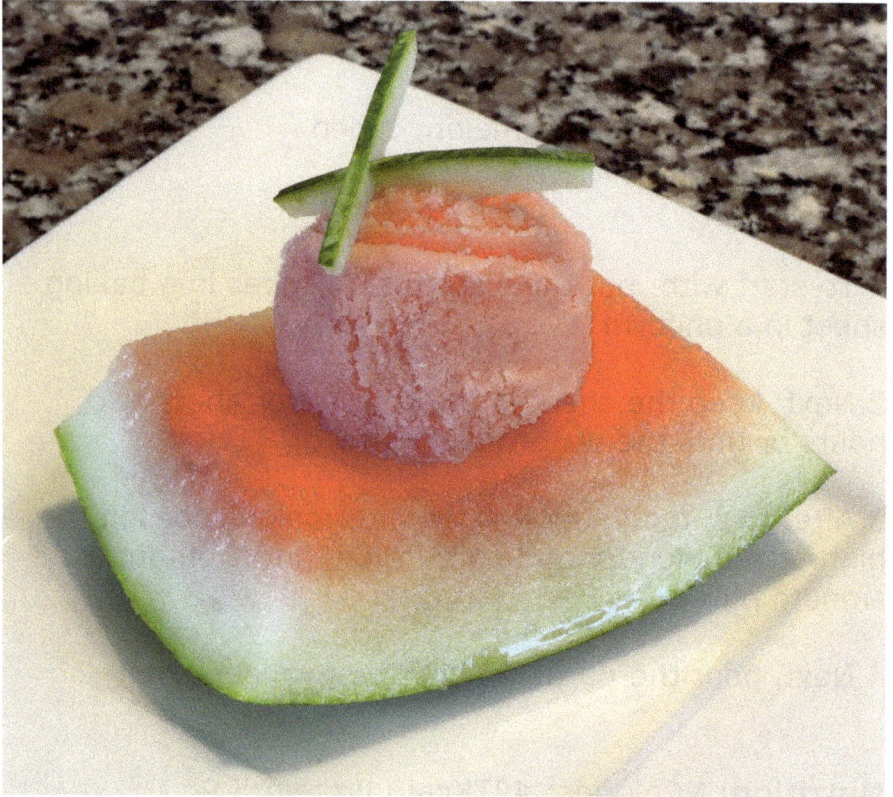

Yummy Fruity Ice-Cream

Prep Time:
20 minutes + 3-4 hours freezing
Cook Time:
0 minutes
Serve: 4

Ingredients:

- ½ cup of coconut cream
- ½ peeled and cut small banana
- 1 cup fresh strawberries, hulled and cut
- 2 tbsp. of shredded coconut

Directions:

1.In a powerful blender, put all together the ingredients and pulse till smooth.

2.Put it into an ice cream maker, then process by the manufacturer's directions.

3.Now, move into an airtight container. Freeze to set for minimum 3- 4 hours, stirring after every thirty minutes.

Nutrition: ‖ Calories: 103 ‖ Fat: 8.2g ‖ Carbohydrates: 8.2g ‖ Protein: 1.2g ‖ Fiber: 2g

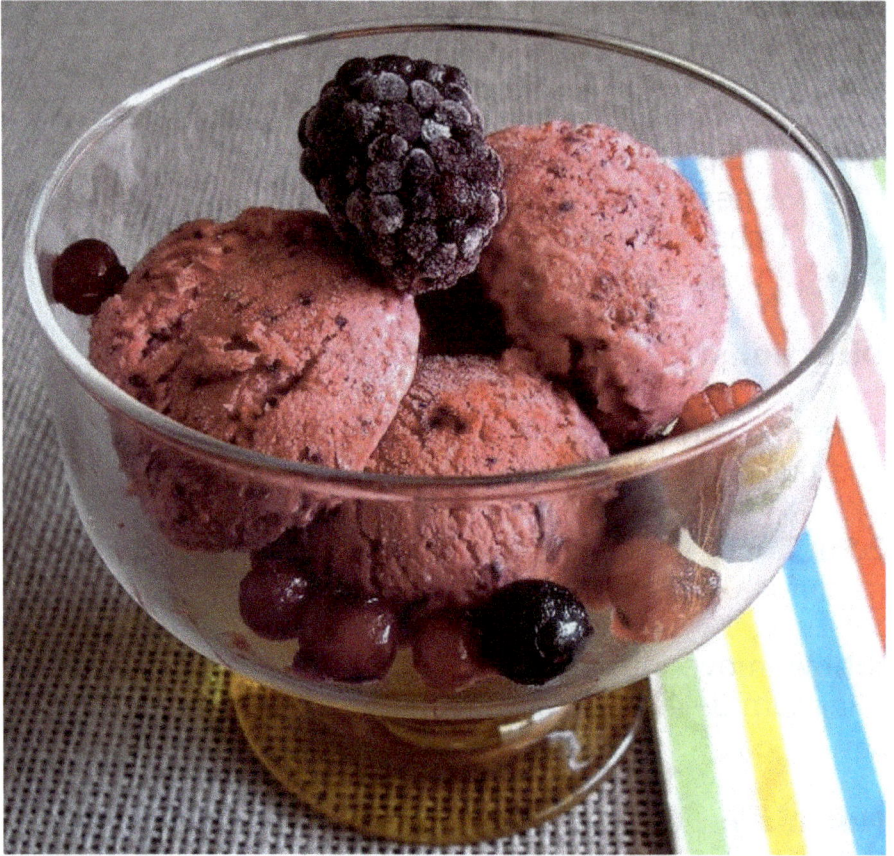

Oregano Dressing on Salad Greens

Prep Time:
15 minutes
Cook Time:
0 minutes
Serve: 4

Ingredients:

- 1/3 cup chopped red onion
- ¾ cup crumbled soft fresh goat cheese
- 1 ½ cups diced celery
- 1 ½ large red bell peppers, diced
- 4 cups baby spinach leaves, coarsely chopped
- 1 tbsp chopped fresh oregano
- 2 tbsp fresh lemon juice
- 2 tbsp extra virgin olive oil

Directions:

1.In a large salad bowl, mix oregano, lemon juice and oil. Add pepper and salt to taste.

2.Mix in red onion, goat cheese, celery, bell peppers and spinach. Toss to coat well, serve and enjoy.

Nutrition: Calories 91, Total Fat 4g, Saturated Fat 0g, Total Carbs 11g, Net Carbs 5g, Protein 6g, Sugar: 3g, Fiber 6g, Sodium 207mg, Potassium 720mg

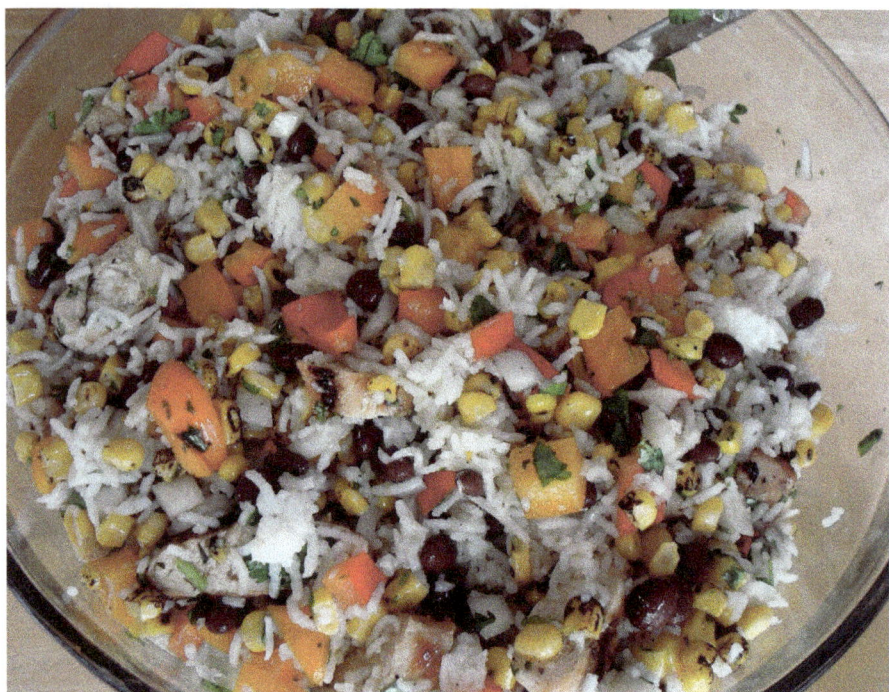

Simple Arugula-Craisins Salad

Prep Time:
10 Minutes
Cook Time:
0 Minutes
Serve: 1

Ingredients:

- 1 cup baby arugula
- 1 cup spinach
- 1 tbsp craisins
- 1 tbsp almonds, shaved or chopped
- 1 tbsp balsamic vinegar
- ½ tbsp extra virgin olive oil

Directions:

1.In a plate, mix arugula and spinach. Top with craisins and almonds. Drizzle olive oil and balsamic vinegar.

Nutrition: Calories 83, Total Fat 4g, Saturated Fat 0g, Total Carbs 11g, Net Carbs 9g, Protein 2g, Sugar: 8g, Fiber 2g, Sodium 93mg, Potassium 273mg

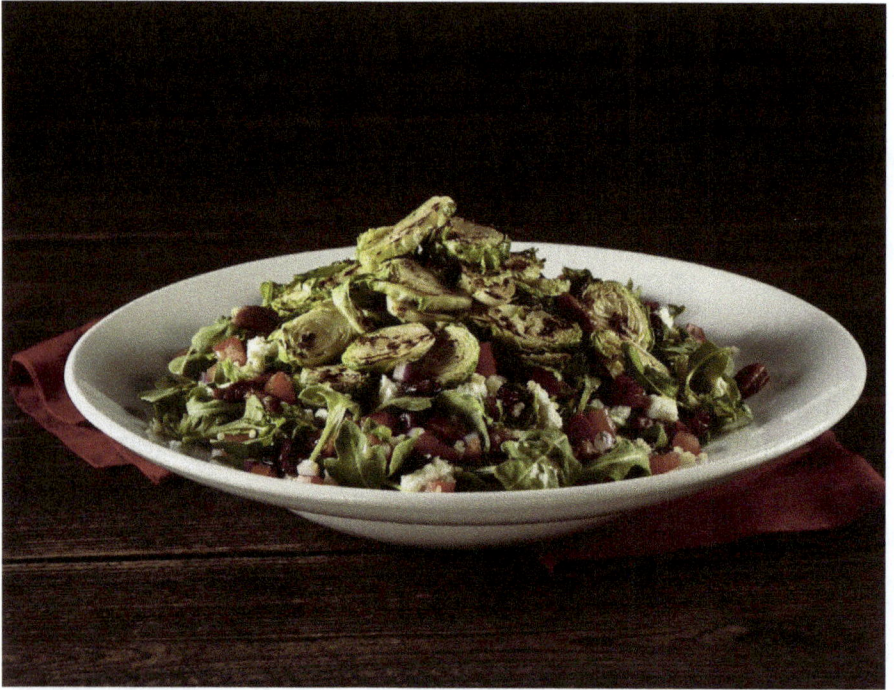

Nutty 'n Warm Brussels Sprouts Salad

Prep Time:
10 Minutes
Cook Time:
10 Minutes
Serve: 4

Ingredients:

- 1 ½ tbsp toasted walnuts, finely chopped
- 1/8 tsp black pepper
- ¼ tsp salt
- ¾ lb. Brussels sprouts
- 1/3 cup fresh breadcrumbs
- 1 garlic clove, minced
- 1 ½ tsp olive oil, divided

Directions:

1.Slice Brussels sprouts in half then separate the leaves from the cores. Cut the cores in quarters and set aside.

2.On medium fire, place a large nonstick saucepan and heat 1 tsp oil. Sauté garlic for a minute.

3.Add breadcrumbs and sauté for another minute or until lightly browned.

4.Transfer to a bowl.

5.In same pan, add remaining oil and cook Brussels sprouts until crisp tender around 8 minutes.

6.Transfer to bowl, pour in breadcrumb mixture and toss to mix.

7.Garnish with nuts before

Nutrition: Calories 71, Total Fat 4g, Saturated Fat 0g, Total Carbs 8g, Net Carbs 4g, Protein 4g, Sugar: 2g, Fiber 4g, Sodium 167mg, Potassium 351mg

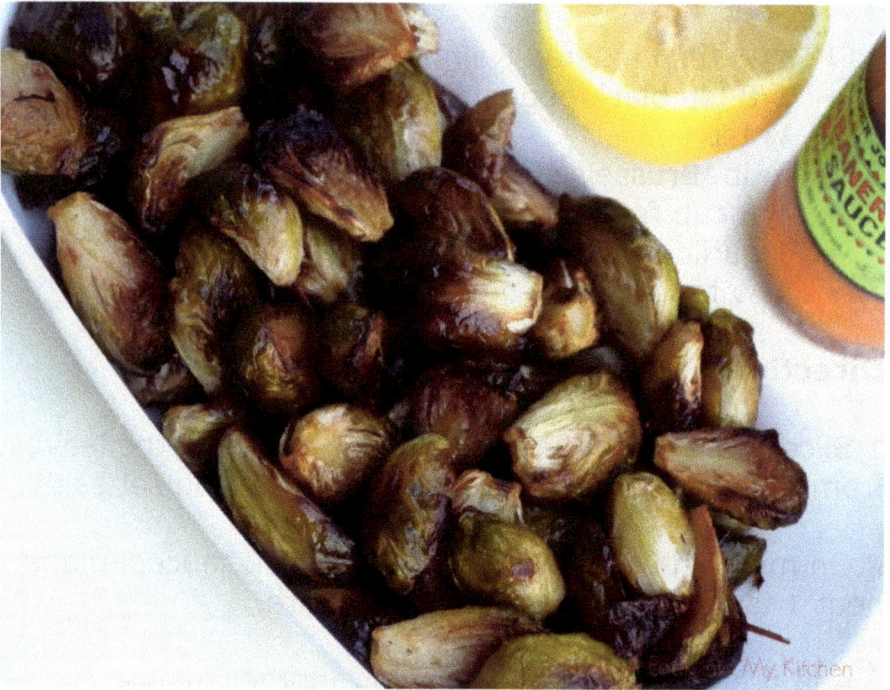

Salad Greens with Roasted Beets

Prep Time:
10 Minutes
Cook Time:
60 Minutes
Serve: 4

Ingredients:

- ½ cup chopped walnuts
- 4 cups baby spinach
- ½ teaspoon Dijon mustard
- 1 tablespoon minced red onions
- 2 tablespoons sherry vinegar
- ¼ cup extra-virgin olive oil
- 3 medium beets, washed and trimmed
- 1 tablespoon dried cranberries, chopped roughly

Directions:

1.In foil, wrap beets and bake in a preheated 400oF oven. Bake until beets are tender, around 1 hour. Once done, open foil and allow to cool. When cool to touch, peel beets and dice.

2.Mix well mustard, red onions, vinegar, and olive oil. Mix in spinach, beets and cranberries. Toss to coat well.

Nutrition: Calories 130, Total Fat 13g, Saturated Fat 1g, Total Carbs 3g, Net Carbs 2g, Protein 3g, Sugar: 1g, Fiber 1g, Sodium 147mg, Potassium 227mg

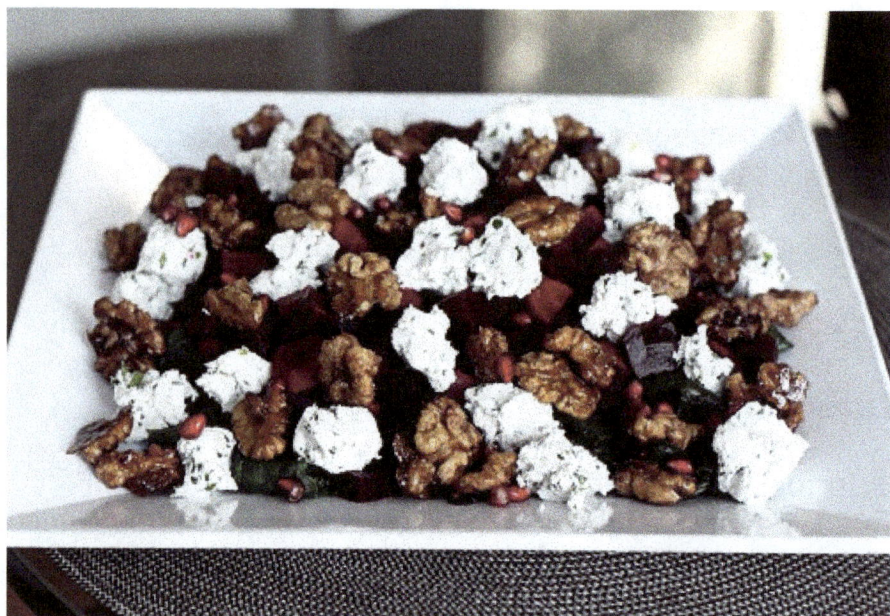

Green Pasta Salad

Prep Time:
15 Minutes
Cook Time:
30 Minutes
Serve: 4

Ingredients:

- 2 cups tubular pasta
- 2 cups green beans, chopped
- 2 cups shredded spinach
- ½ cup parmesan cheese
- 3 cloves of garlic
- Salt to taste
- 4 tablespoons olive oil

Directions:

1.Cook the pasta according to package instructions. Drain then set aside.

2.Heat a little olive oil in a skillet over medium heat and add the green beans and garlic.

3.Sauté for 3 to 5 minutes.

4.Toss the pasta together with the sautéed green beans and garlic.

5.Add in the spinach and parmesan cheese. Season with salt. Toss to coat.

Nutrition: Calories: 280; Fat: 18g; Carbs: 25g; Protein: 7g

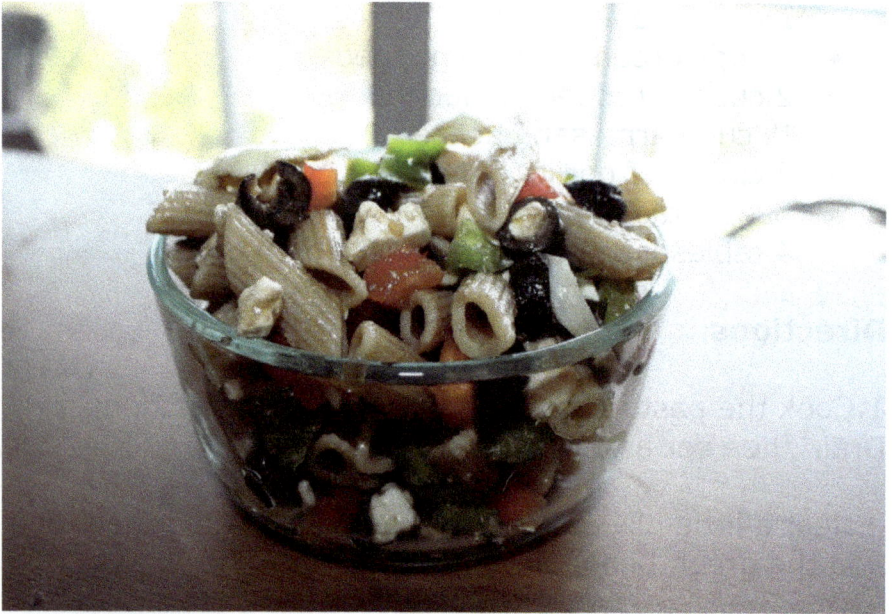

Tomato, Peach, And Burrata Salad

Prep Time:
5 Minutes
Cook Time:
15 Minutes
Serve: 4

Ingredients:

- 1/3 cup balsamic vinegar
- 2 large tomatoes, cut into piece
- 2 large peaches, pitted and cut into pieces
- 6 ounces burrata cheese, cut into cubes
- 3 tablespoons chopped basil
- Salt to taste

Directions:

1. Make balsamic reduction by boiling the balsamic vinegar over low heat for 15 minutes. Remove from the heat and set aside.

2. Arrange the tomatoes, peaches, and cheese on a platter.

3. Drizzle with balsamic reduction and season with salt to taste. Garnish with basil.

Nutrition: Calories: 197; Fat: 11g; Carbs: 17g; Protein: 9g

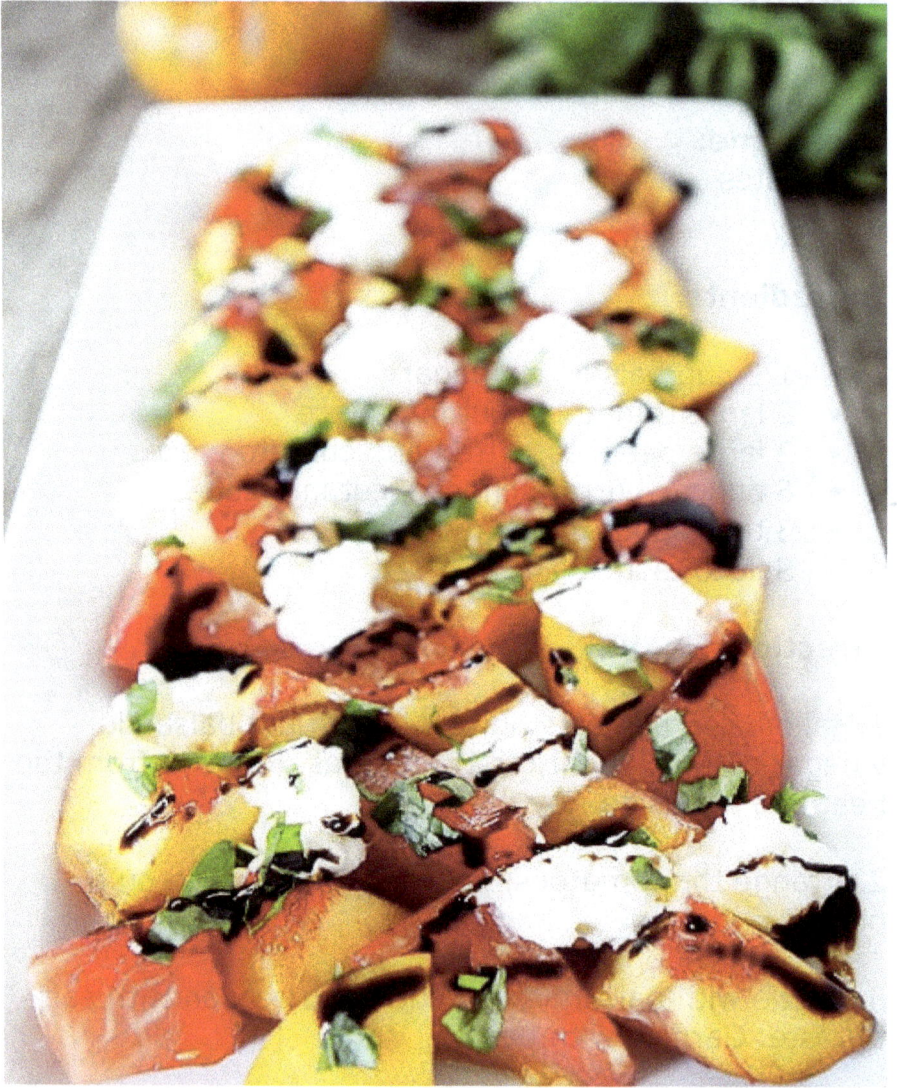

Watermelon and Cucumber Salad

Prep Time:
10 Minutes
Cook Time:
0 Minutes
Serve: 10

Ingredients:

- ½ large watermelon, diced
- 1 cucumber, peeled and diced
- 1 red onion, chopped
- ¼ cup feta cheese
- ½ cup balsamic vinegar
- Salt to taste

Directions:

1.Place all ingredients in a bowl. Toss everything to coat.

2.Place in the fridge to cool before.

Nutrition: Calories: 24; Fat: 0g; Carbs: 3g; Protein: 0.8g

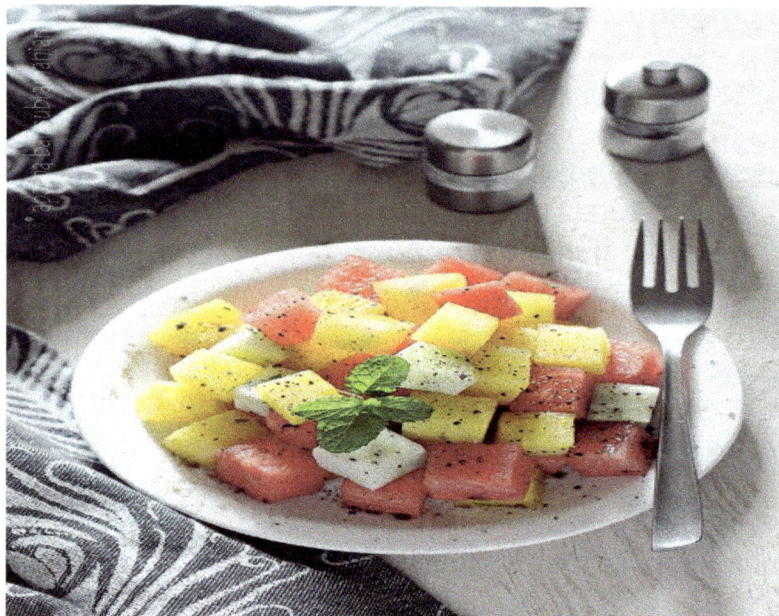

Pasta Salad

Prep Time:
5 Minutes
Cook Time:
10 Minutes
Serve: 4

Ingredients:

- 1-pound dry whole wheat pasta
- ¾ cup red peppers, seeded and chopped
- ¾ cup commercial basil pesto
- 1 small mozzarella cheese ball, diced
- 3 handfuls of arugulas, washed
- Water for boiling
- Salt and pepper to taste

Directions:

1.Boil water in a stock pot and cook the pasta according to package instructions. Drain and allow to cool.

2.Mix all ingredients in a salad bowl and toss to coat.

3.Season with salt and pepper to taste.

Nutrition: Calories: 461; Fat: 6g; Carbs: 88g; Protein: 20g

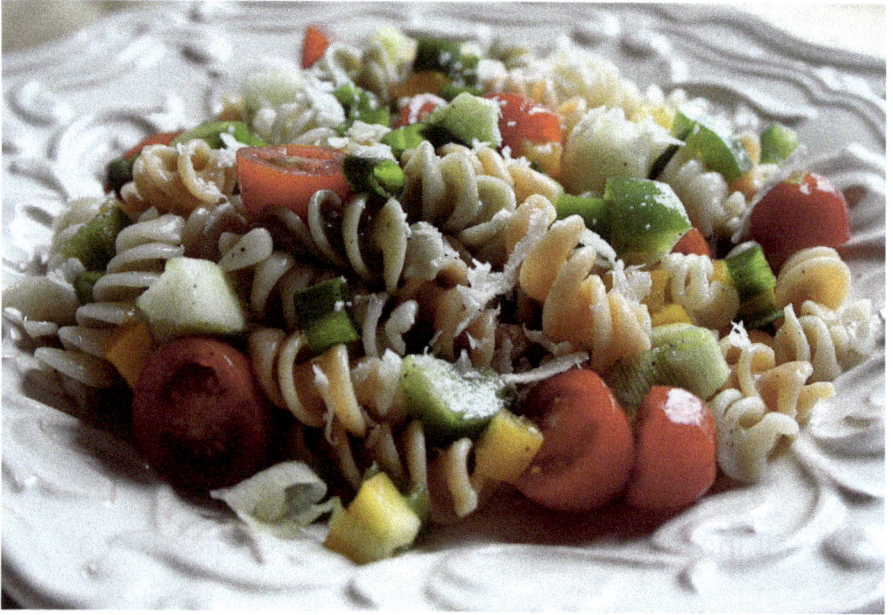

Marinated Kale Salad

Prep Time:
10 Minutes
Cook Time:
0 Minutes
Serve: 2

Ingredients:

- 1 bunch curly kale, washed and torn
- 1 tablespoon almond butter
- 2 1/2 tablespoons apple cider vinegar
- 2 tablespoons liquid aminos or soy sauce
- 1 tablespoon agave nectar or honey

Directions:

1.Place all ingredients in a container.

2.Allow to marinate in the fridge for at least 10 minutes before.

Nutrition: Calories: 114; Fat: 5g; Carbs: 16g; Protein: 4g

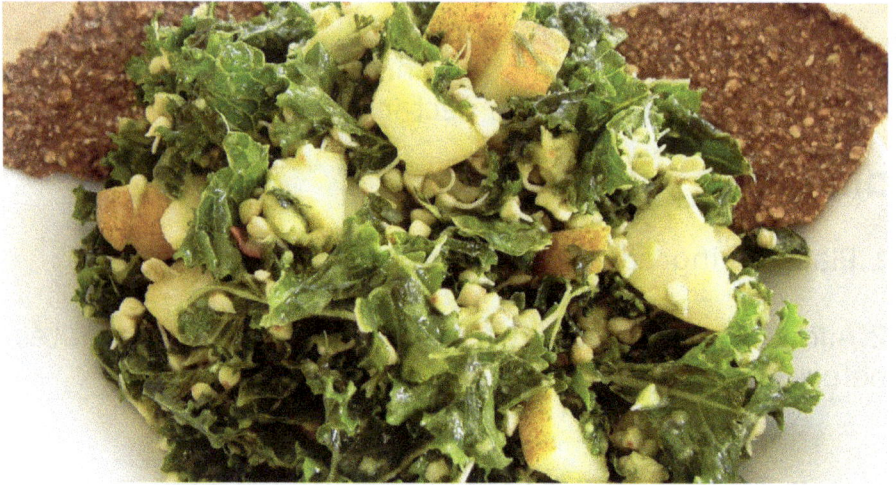

Israeli Salad Recipe

Prep Time:
10 Minutes
Cook Time:
0 Minutes
 Serve: 4

Ingredients:

- 2 cups diced cherry tomatoes
- 2 cups cucumber, diced
- ¼ cup red onion, sliced
- ¼ cup chopped mint
- 2 tablespoons olive oil
- Salt to taste
- 1 tablespoon lemon juice

Directions:

1.Place all ingredients in salad bowl.

2.Toss to mix everything.

3.Place inside the fridge to chill.

Nutrition: Calories: 81; Fat: 6g; Carbs: 8g; Protein: 1g

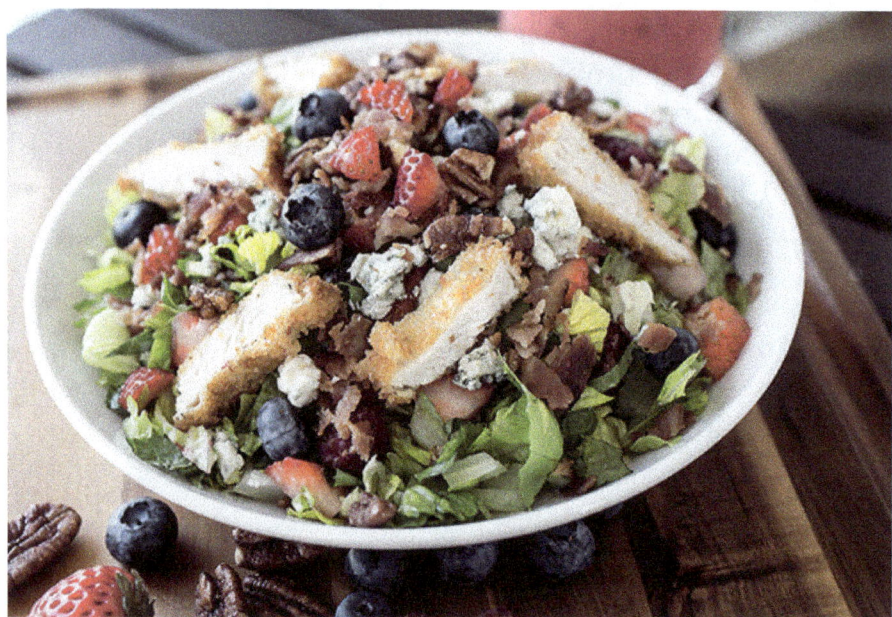

Strawberry, Cucumber, And Mozzarella Salad

Prep Time:
10 Minutes
Cook Time:
0 Minutes
Serve: 3

Ingredients:

- 5 ounces organic salad greens of your choice
- 2 medium cucumber, spiralized
- 2 cups strawberries, hulled and chopped
- 8 ounces mini mozzarella cheese balls
- ½ cup balsamic vinegar
- Salt to taste

Directions:

1.Toss all ingredients in a salad bowl.

2.Allow to chill in the fridge for at least 10 minutes before.

Nutrition: Calories: 287; Fat: 21g; Carbs: 14g; Protein: 11g

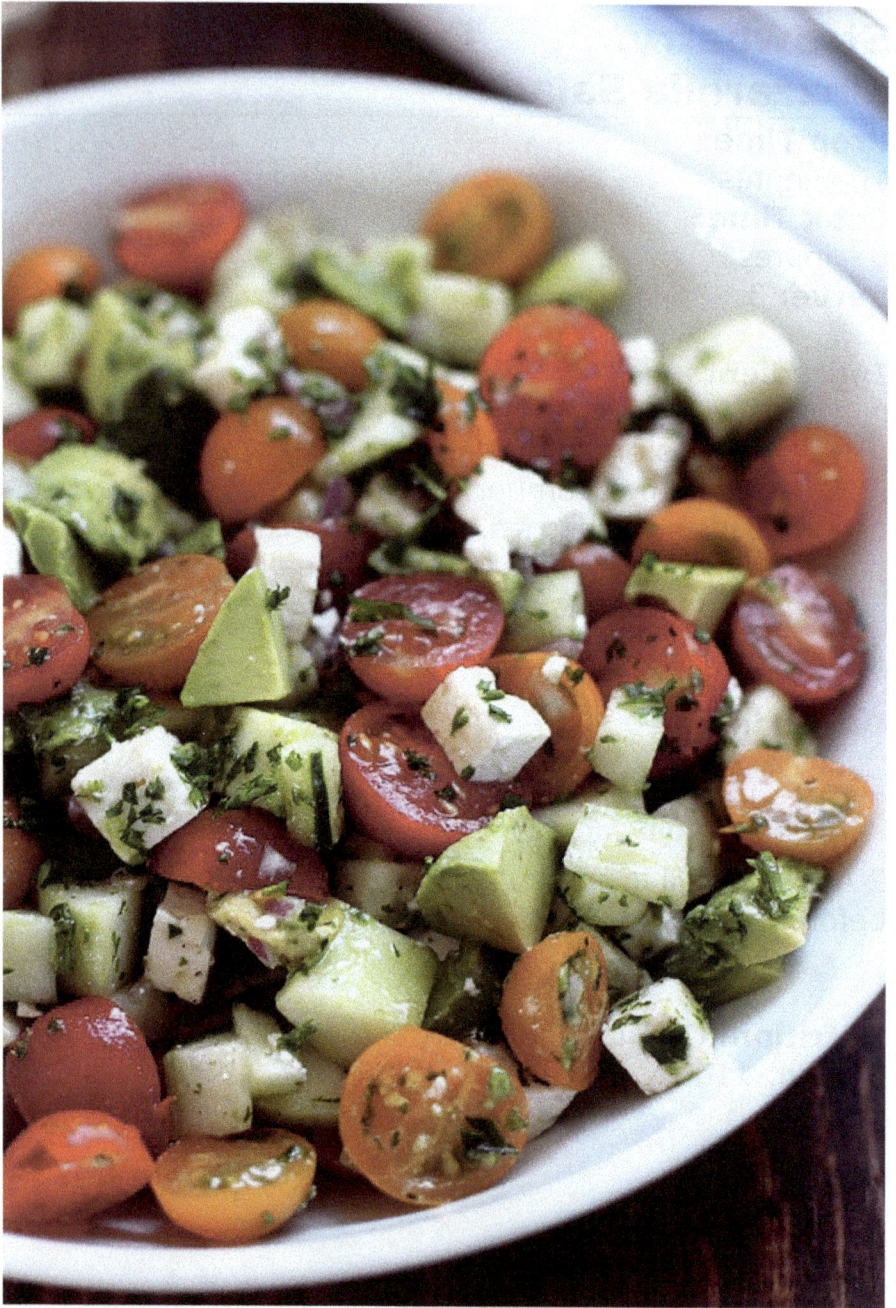

Citrusy Brussels Sprouts Salad

Prep Time:
15 Minutes
Cook Time:
3 Minutes
Serve: 6

Ingredients:

- 2 tablespoons olive oil
- 1-pound Brussels sprouts
- 1 cup walnuts
- Juice from 1 lemon
- ½ cup grated parmesan cheese
- Salt and pepper to taste

Directions:

1.Heat oil in a skillet over medium flame and sauté the Brussels sprouts for 3 minutes until slightly wilted. Removed from heat and allow to cool.

2.In a bowl, toss together the cooled Brussels sprouts and the rest of the ingredients. Toss to coat.

Nutrition: Calories: 259; Fat: 23g; Carbs: 12g; Protein: 6g

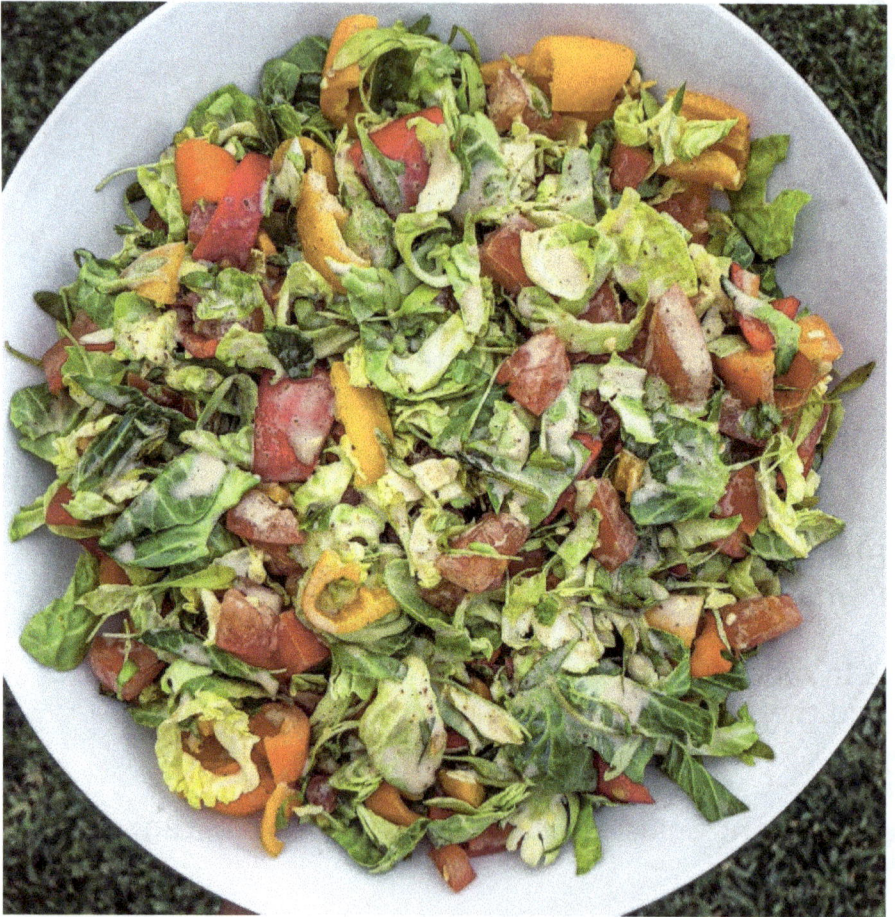

Crunchy and Salty Cucumber Salad

Prep Time:
10 Minutes
Cook Time:
0 Minutes
Serve: 4

Ingredients:

- 2 candy-striped (Chioggiabeets, trimmed and peeled
- 2 Persian cucumbers, sliced thinly
- 1 medium radish, trimmed and sliced thinly
- Juice from 1 lemon
- ½ cup parmesan cheese, shredded
- A dash of flaky sea salt
- A dash of ground black pepper Olive oil for drizzling

Directions:

1.Place all vegetables in a bowl.

2.Stir in the lemon juice and parmesan cheese.

3.Season with salt and pepper to taste

3.Add olive oil or salad oil. Toss to mix everything.

Nutrition: Calories: 71; Fat: 4g; Carbs: 6g; Protein: 4g

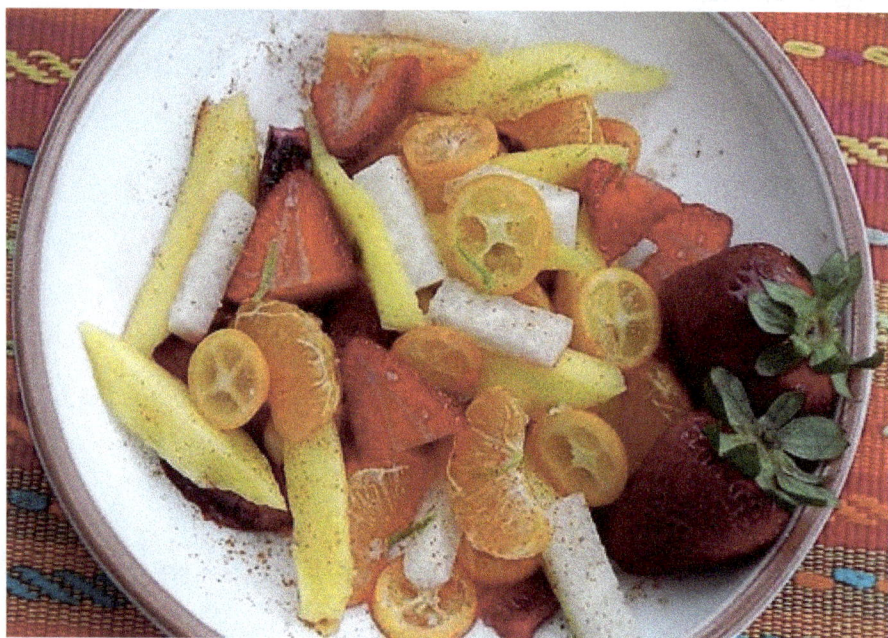

Celery Salad

Prep Time:
5 Minutes
Cook Time:
0 Minutes
Serve: 4

Ingredients:

- 3 cups celery, thinly sliced
- ½ cup parmigiana cheese, shaved
- 1/3 cup toasted walnuts
- 3 tablespoons extra virgin olive oil
- 1 tablespoon red wine vinegar
- Salt and pepper to taste

Directions:

1.Place the celery, cheese, and walnuts in a bowl.

2.In a smaller bowl, combine the olive oil and vinegar. Season with salt and pepper to taste. Whisk to combine everything.

3.Drizzle over the celery, cheese, and walnuts. Toss to coat.

Nutrition: Calories: 142; Fat: 4g; Carbs: 13g; Protein: 4

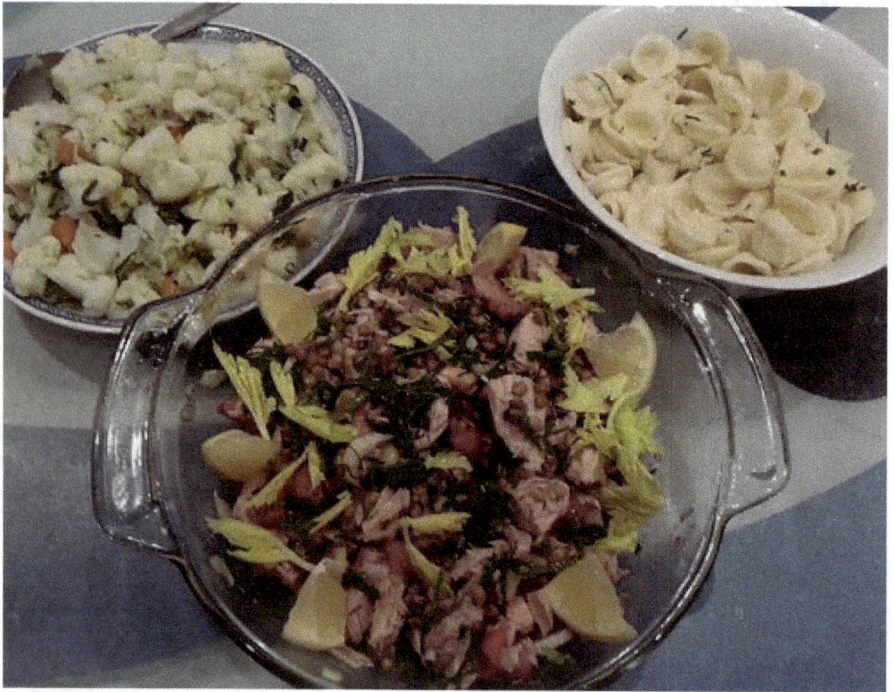

Grilled Corn Salad with Feta Cheese

Prep Time:
5 Minutes
Cook Time:
15 Minutes
Serve: 6

Ingredients:

- 6 large ears of corn, peeled and hulled
- ¼ cup chopped red onion
- ½ cup Feta cheese, crumbled
- 2 tablespoon extra-virgin olive oil
- Chopped mint for garnish
- Salt and pepper to taste

Directions:

1.Heat the grill to medium high and grill the corn for 12 minutes.

2.Cut the kernels off the cob and place on a bowl.

3.Add the rest of the ingredients and toss to mix everything.

Nutrition: Calories: 153; Fat: 8g; Carbs: 18g; Protein: 5g

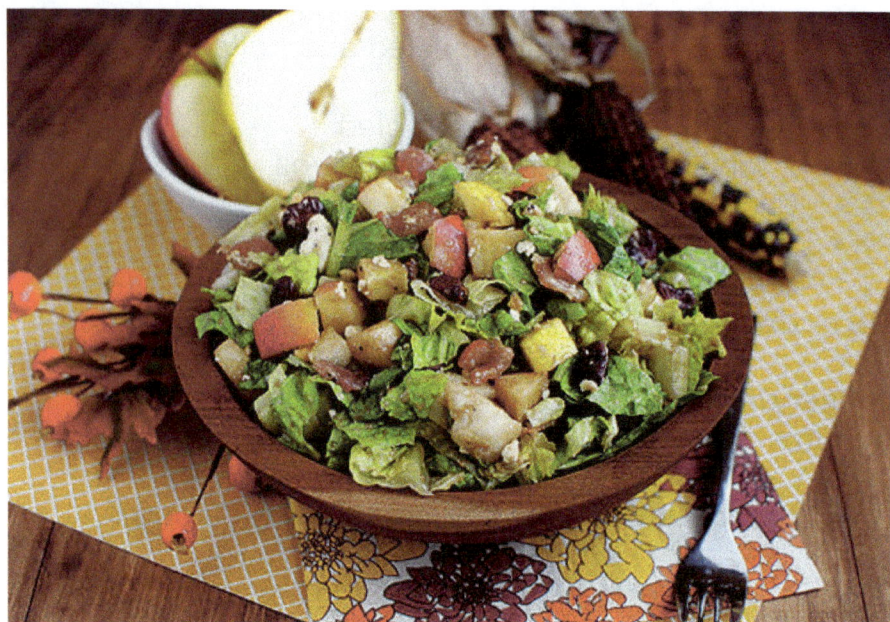

Pear and Pomegranate Salsa

Prep Time:
10 Minutes
Cook Time:
0 Minutes
Serve: 3

Ingredients:

- 2 fresh pears, cored and diced
- Seeds from 1 fresh pomegranate
- ½ onion, diced
- ½ cup fresh cilantro leaves, chopped
- Juice from ½ lime
- Salt and pepper to taste

Directions:

1.Toss all ingredients in a bowl to combine. Serve immediately.

2.Best served with grilled meats.

Nutrition: Calories: 122; Fat: 1g; Carbs: 29g; Protein:2 g

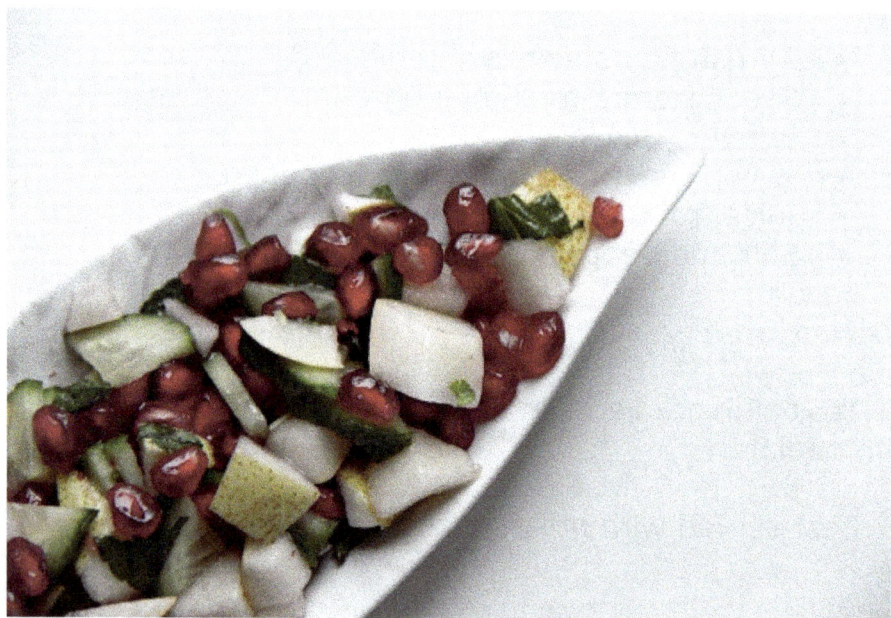

Lentil Tomato Salad

Prep Time:
5 Minutes
Cook Time:
0 Minutes
Serve: 4

Ingredients:

- 15 ounces canned lentils, rinsed and drained
- 1 ½ cups cherry tomatoes, sliced
- ¼ cup white wine vinegar
- 1/8 cup chives
- 1 tablespoon olive oil Salt and pepper to taste

Directions:

1.Put all ingredients in a bowl. Toss to combine.

Nutrition: Calories: 231; Fat: 12g; Carbs: 23g;
Protein: 10g

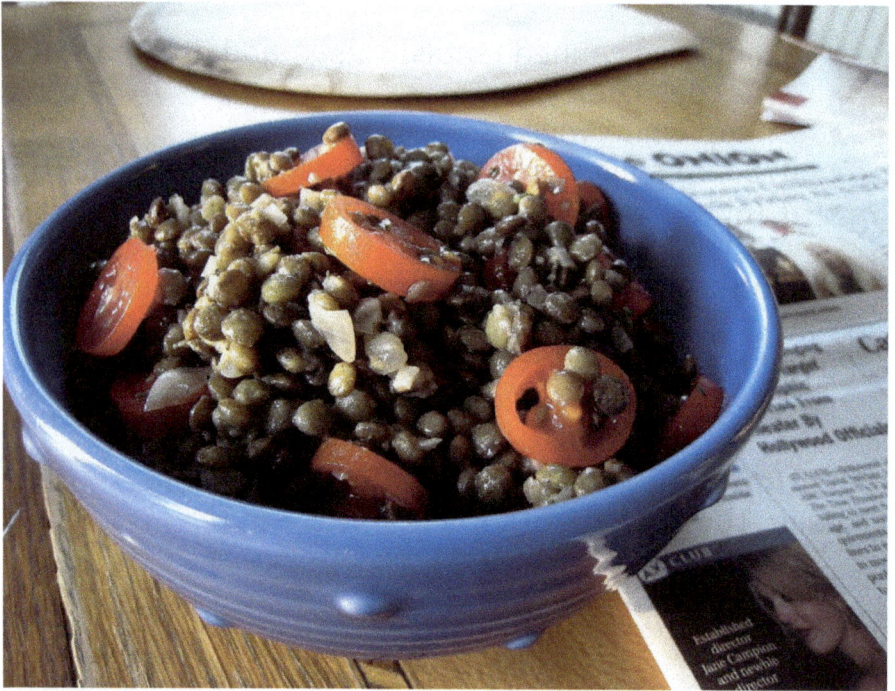

Asparagus Niçoise Salad

Prep Time:
20 Minutes
Cook Time:
20 Minutes
Serve: 4

Ingredients:

- 1-pound small red potatoes, cleaned and halved
- 1-pound fresh asparagus, trimmed and halved
- 2 ½ ounces white tuna in water
- ½ cup pitted Greek olives, halved
- ½ cup zesty Italian salad dressing
- Water for boiling
- Salt and pepper to taste

Directions:

1.Boil water in a stockpot over medium flame.

2.Put in the potatoes and cook for 20 minutes or the potatoes are tender. Blanch the asparagus for 3 minutes and set aside.

3.Place all ingredients in a bowl. Toss to mix all ingredients.

Nutrition: Calories: 223; Fat: 8g; Carbs: 23g; Protein: 16g

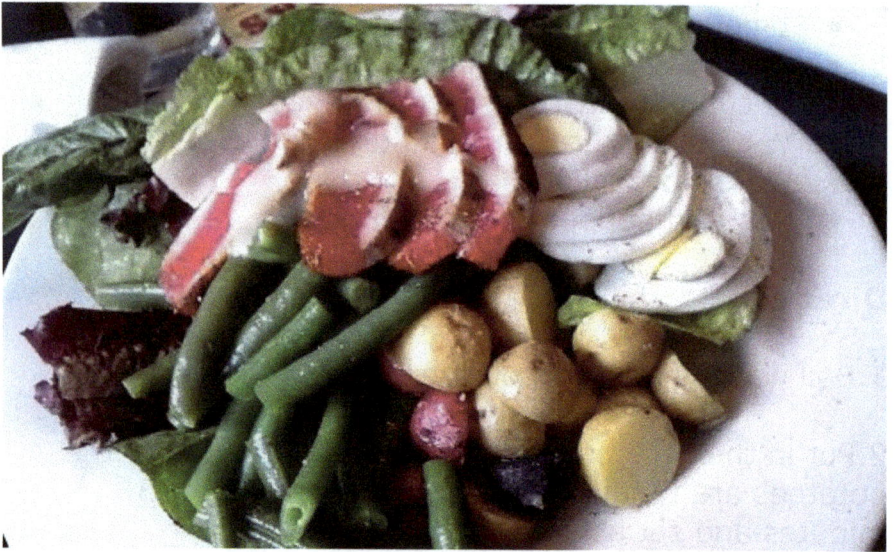

Bacon and Pea Salad

Prep Time:
10 Minutes
Cook Time:
5 Minutes
Serve: 6

Ingredients:

- 4 bacon strips
- 4 cups fresh peas
- ½ cup shredded cheddar cheese
- ½ cup ranch salad dressing
- 1/3 cup chopped red onions
- Salt and pepper to taste

Directions:

1.Heat skillet over medium flame and fry the bacon until crispy or until the fat has rendered.

2.Transfer into a plate lined with paper towel and crumble.

3.In a bowl, combine the rest of the ingredients and toss to coat.

4.Add in the bacon bits last.

Nutrition: Calories: 218; Fat: 14g; Carbs: 14g; Protein: 9g

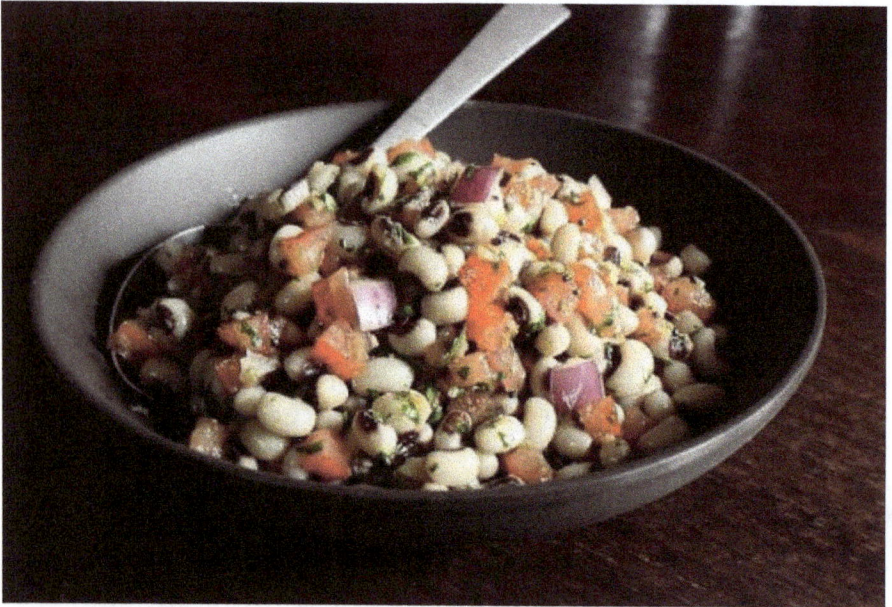

Insalata Caprese

Prep Time:
10 Minutes
Cook Time:
0 Minutes
Serve: 8

Ingredients:

- 2 ½ pounds tomatoes, cut into 1-inch pieces
- 8 ounces mozzarella cheese pearls
- ½ cup ripe olives, pitted
- ¼ cup fresh basil, sliced thinly
- Balsamic vinegar
- Optional Salt and pepper to taste
- 3 tablespoons olive oil

Directions:

1.Place all ingredients in a bowl.

2.Season with salt and pepper to taste.

3.Drizzle with balsamic vinegar if available.

4.Toss to coat.

Nutrition: Calories: 160; Fat: 12g; Carbs: 7g; Protein: 6g

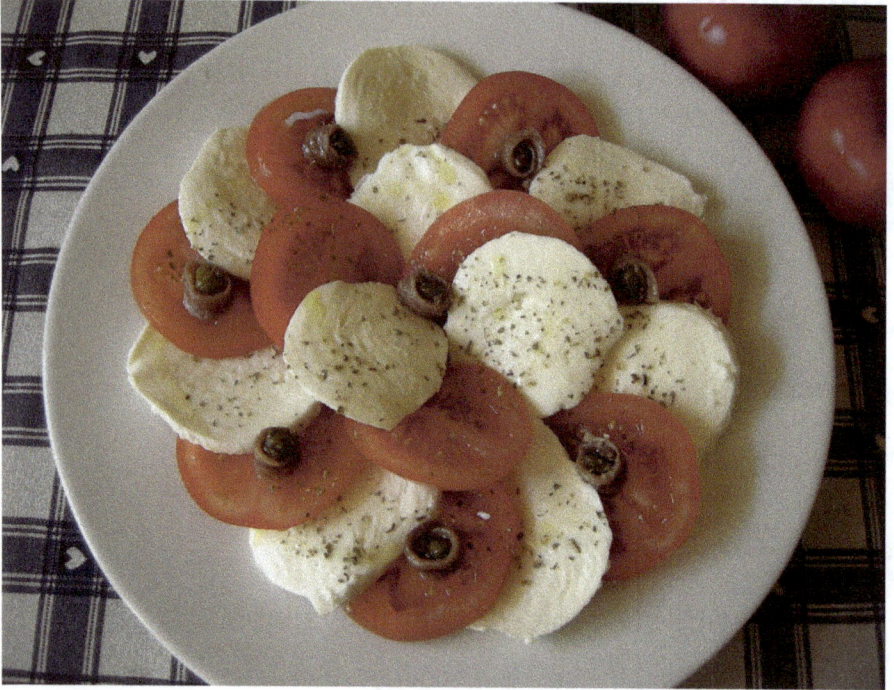

Salmon Salad with Walnuts

Prep Time:
10 Minutes
Cook Time:
10 Minutes
Serve: 2

Ingredients:

- 2 salmon fillets
- 6 tablespoons balsamic vinaigrette,
- divided 1/8 teaspoon pepper
- 4 cups mixed salad greens
- 1/4 cup walnuts
- 2 tablespoons crumbled cheese
- Salt and pepper to taste

Directions:

1. Brush the salmon with half of the balsamic vinaigrette and sprinkle with pepper.

2. Grill the salmon over medium heat for 5 minutes on each side.

3. Crumble the salmon and place in a mixing bowl.

4. Add the rest of the ingredients and season with salt and pepper to taste.

Nutrition: Calories: 374; Fat: 25g; Carbs: 13g; Protein: 24g

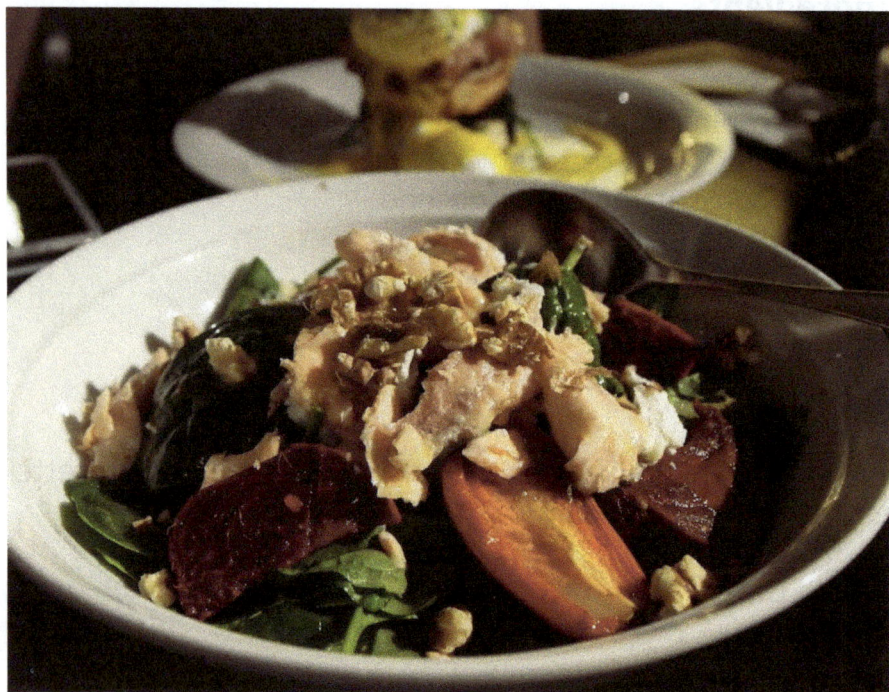

Salmon White Bean Spinach Salad

Prep Time:
10 Minutes
Cook Time:
10 Minutes
Serve: 4

Ingredients:

- 4 salmon fillets
- 15 ounces great northern beans, rinsed and drained
- ½ cup commercial vinaigrette of your choice
- 11 ounces baby spinach
- 1 red onion, cut into thin slices
- Salt and pepper to taste

Directions:

1.Season the salmon fillets with salt and pepper.

2.Place in a baking pan and bake for 4000F for 10 minutes or until the fish becomes flaky. Cool slightly.

3.In a large bowl, toss the beans and vinaigrette. Toss in the spinach and onions.

4.Divide the salad among four plates and top with salmon.

Nutrition: Calories: 577; Fat: 17; Carbs: 26; Protein: 76g

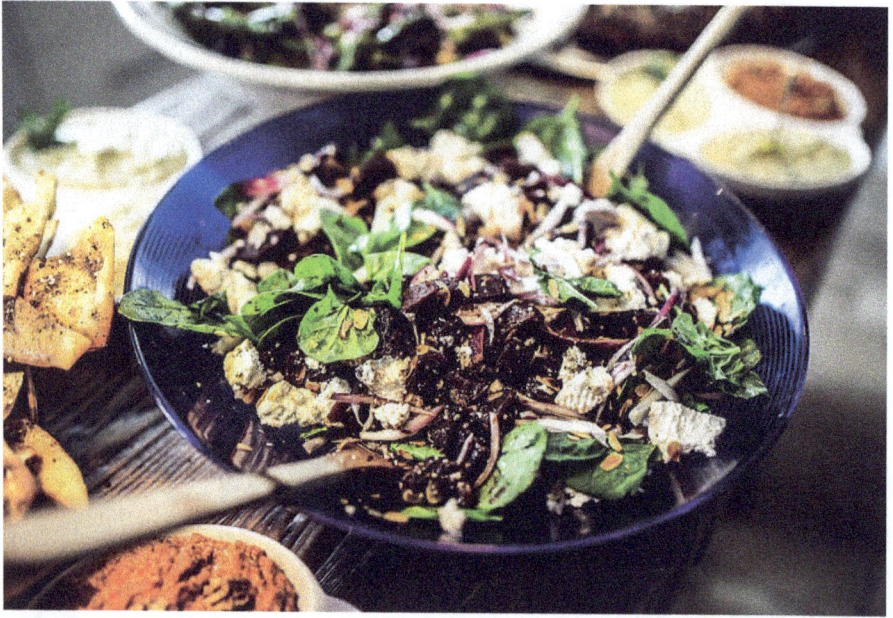

Balsamic Cucumber Salad

Prep Time:
10 Minutes
Cook Time:
 0 Minutes
Serve: 6

Ingredients:

- 1 large English cucumber, halved and sliced
- 2 cups grape tomatoes, halved
- 1 medium red onion, sliced thinly
- ½ cup balsamic vinaigrette
- ¾ cup feta cheese
- Salt and pepper to taste

Directions:

1. Place all ingredients in a bowl.

2. Toss to coat everything with the dressing.

3. Allow to chill before.

Nutrition: Calories: 90; Fat: 5g; Carbs: 9g; Protein: 4g

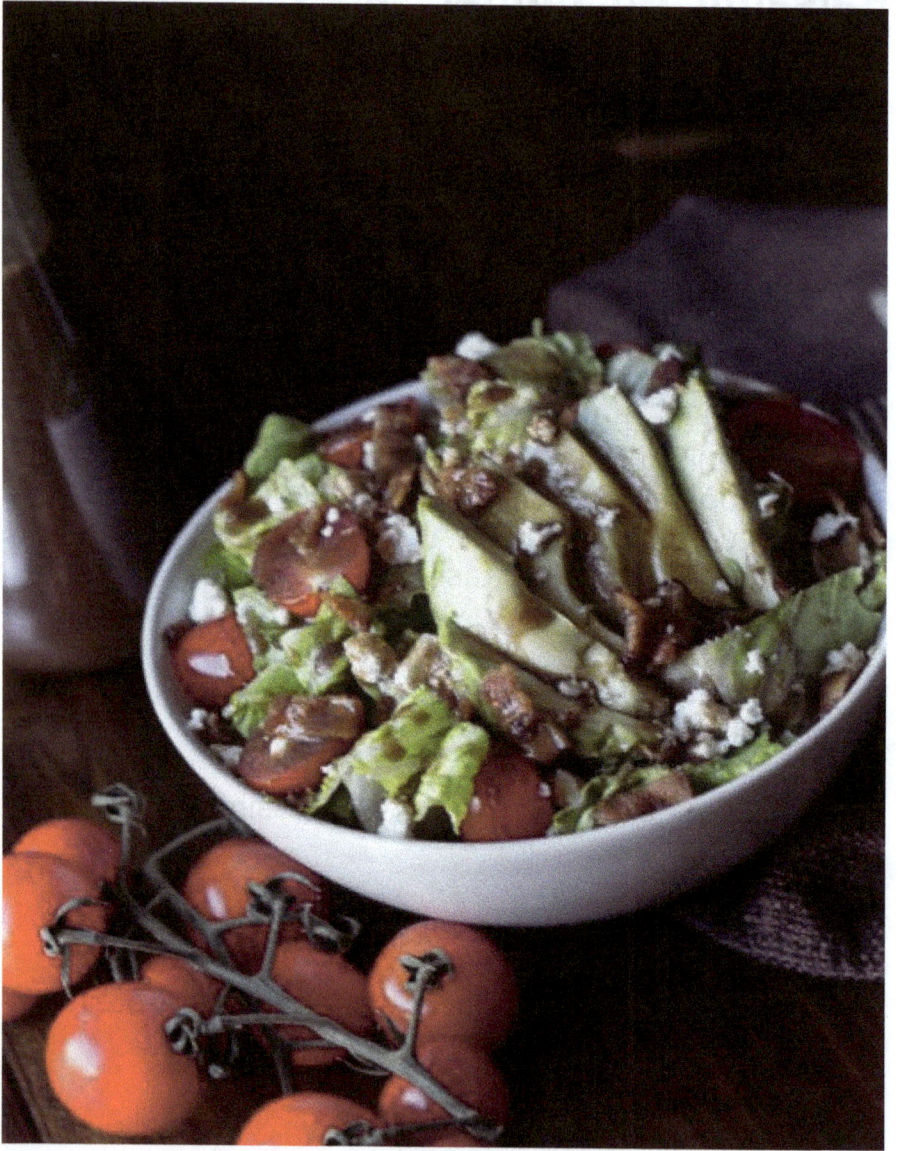

Sour Cream and Cucumbers

Prep Time:
15 Minutes
Cook Time:
0 Minutes
Serve: 8

Ingredients:

- ½ cup sour cream
- 3 tablespoons white vinegar
- 1 tablespoon sugar
- 4 medium cucumbers, sliced thinly
- 1 small sweet onion, sliced thinly
- Salt and pepper to taste

Directions:

1.In a bowl, whisk the sour cream, vinegar, and sugar.

2.Season with salt and pepper to taste. Whisk until well-combined.

3.Add in the cucumber and the rest of the ingredients. Toss to coat.

4.Allow to chill before.

Nutrition: Calories: 62; Fat: 3g; Carbs: 7g; Protein: 2g

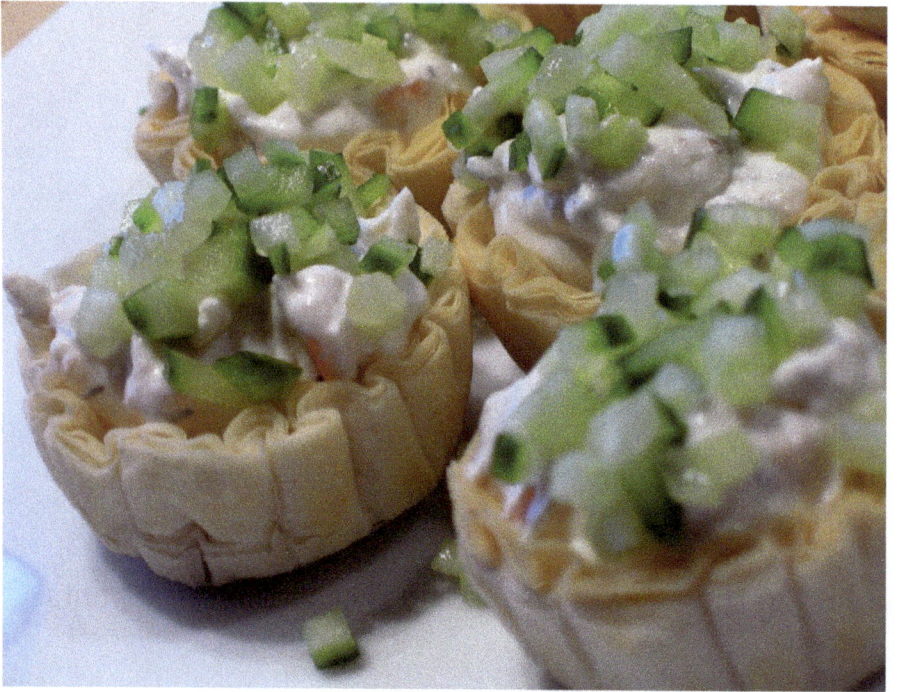

Minty Watermelon Cucumber Salad

Prep Time:
10 Minutes
Cook Time:
0 Minutes
Serve: 12

Ingredients:

- 8 cups cubed seedless watermelon
- 2 English cucumbers, halved and sliced
- ¼ cup minced fresh mint
- ¼ cup balsamic vinegar
- ¼ cup olive oil
- Salt and pepper to taste

Directions:

1.Place everything in a bowl and toss to coat everything.

2.Allow to chill before.

Nutrition: Calories: 60; Fat: 3g; Carbs: 9g; Protein: 1g

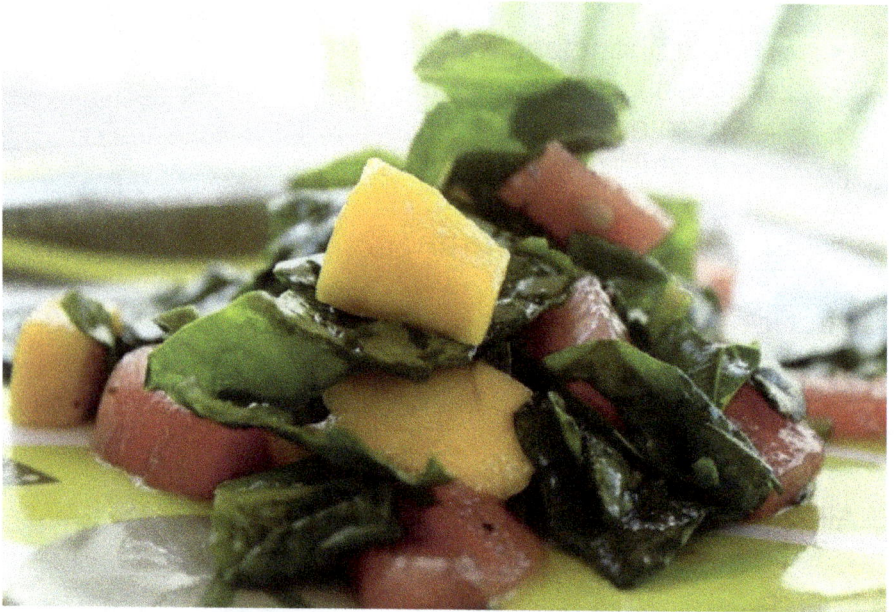

Easy Kale Salad

Prep Time:
10 Minutes
Cook Time:
0 Minutes
Serve: 8

Ingredients:

- 10 cups kale, sliced thinly
- 1 apple, thinly sliced
- 3 tablespoons olive oil
- 2 tablespoons lemon juice
- ¼ cup crumbled feta cheese
- Salt and pepper to taste

Directions:

1.Place kale in a bowl and massage kale until the leaves become soft and darkened.

2.Add in the apples.

3.In another bowl, whisk the oil, lemon juice, salt, and pepper.

4.Drizzle the sauce over the kale and sprinkle with cheese on top.

Nutrition: Calories: 113; Fat: 9g; Carbs: 6g; Protein: 4g

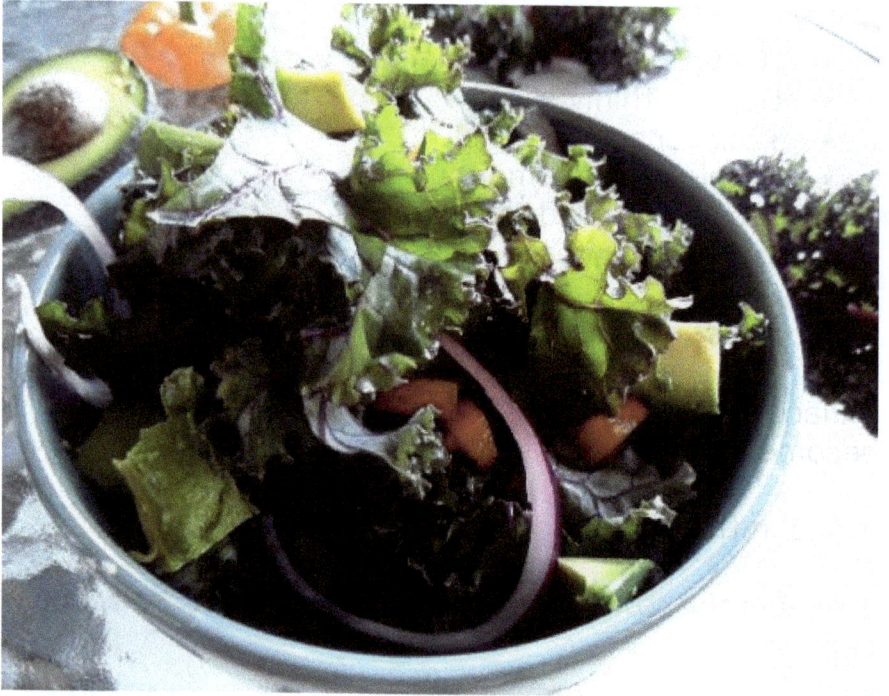

Pear Blue Cheese Salad

Prep Time:
10 Minutes
Cook Time:
0 Minutes
Serve: 10

Ingredients:

- 12 cups romaine lettuce, torn
- 2/3 cup balsamic vinegar
- 2 medium pears, sliced
- 2/3 cup crumbled blue cheese
- 2/3 cup glazed pecans
- Salt and pepper to taste

Directions:

1.Toss all ingredients in a bowl to combine.

2.Allow to chill before.

Nutrition: Calories: 133; Fat: 8g; Carbs: 12g; Protein: 3g

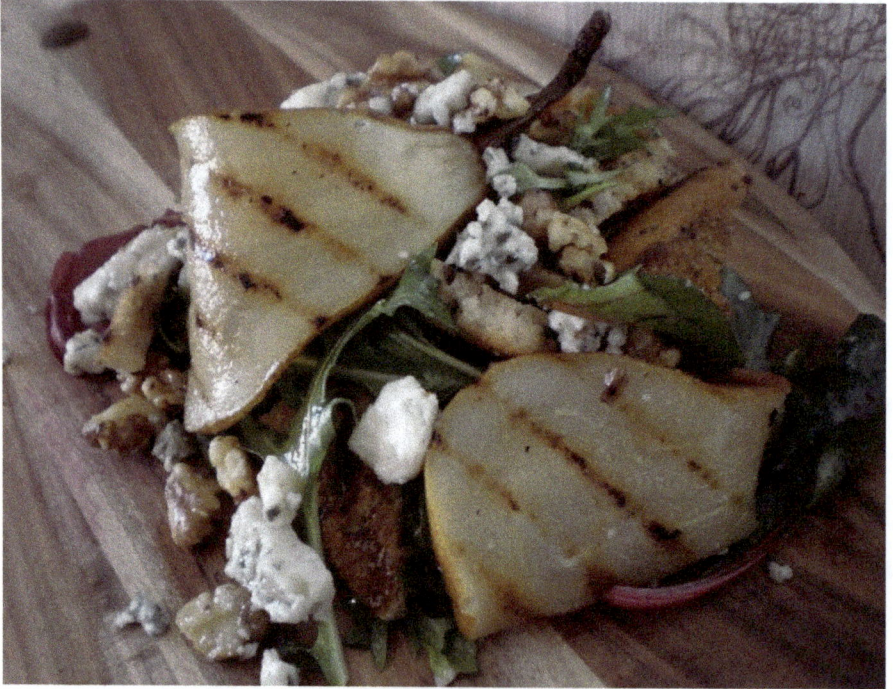

Salad Greens with Garlic Maple Salad

Prep Time:
10 Minutes
Cook Time:
0 Minutes
Serve: 4

Ingredients:

- 2 pounds mixed salad greens, washed
- 1/3 cup olive oil
- ¼ cup maple syrup
- 3 cloves of garlic, minced
- Juice from 1 lemon
- Salt and pepper to taste

Directions:

1.Place the salad greens in a bowl.

2.In a smaller bowl, combine the olive oil, maple syrup, garlic, and lemon juice.

3.Season with salt and pepper to taste.

4.Drizzle over the salad greens and toss.

Nutrition: Calories: 145; Fat:12 g; Carbs: 10g; Protein: 1g

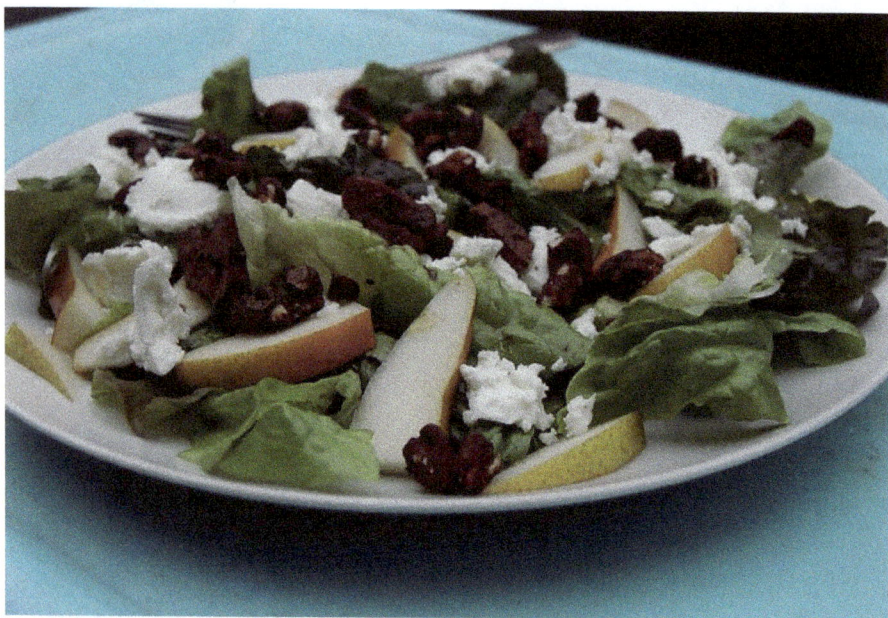

Citrus Avocado Spinach Salad

Prep Time:
10 Minutes
Cook Time:
0 Minutes
Serve: 8

Ingredients:

- 8 cups baby spinach; washed and drained
- 3 cups orange segments, seeded and halved
- 2 medium ripe avocadoes, peeled and sliced
- 1 cup blue cheese, crumbled
- Salad dressing of your choice
- Salt and pepper to taste

Directions:

1.Place the spinach, oranges, and avocado slices in a bowl.

2.Add in the cheese and drizzle with the salad dressing of your choice. Toss to coat everything.

Nutrition: Calories: 168; Fat:10g; Carbs: 16g; Protein: 5g

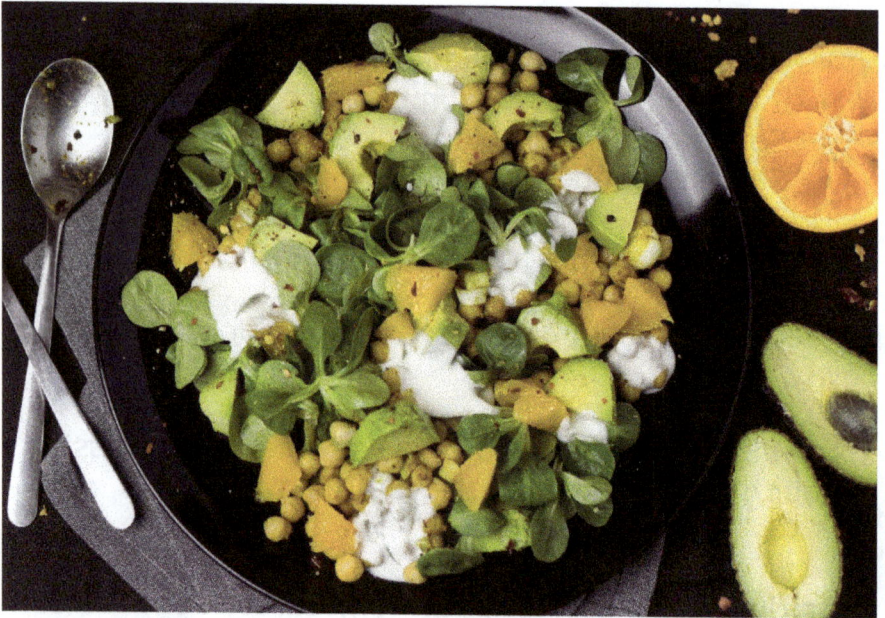

Kale And Brussels Sprouts Salad

Prep Time:
10 Minutes
Cook Time:
 0 Minutes
Serve: 6

Ingredients:

- 1 small bunch kale, thinly sliced
- ½ pound fresh Brussels sprouts, thinly sliced
- ½ cup pistachios, chopped coarsely
- ½ cup honey mustard salad dressing
- ¼ cup parmesan cheese, shredded
- Salt and pepper to taste

Directions:

1.Place all ingredients in a salad bowl.

2.Toss to coat everything.

Nutrition: Calories: 207; Fat: 14g; Carbs: 16g;
Protein: 7g

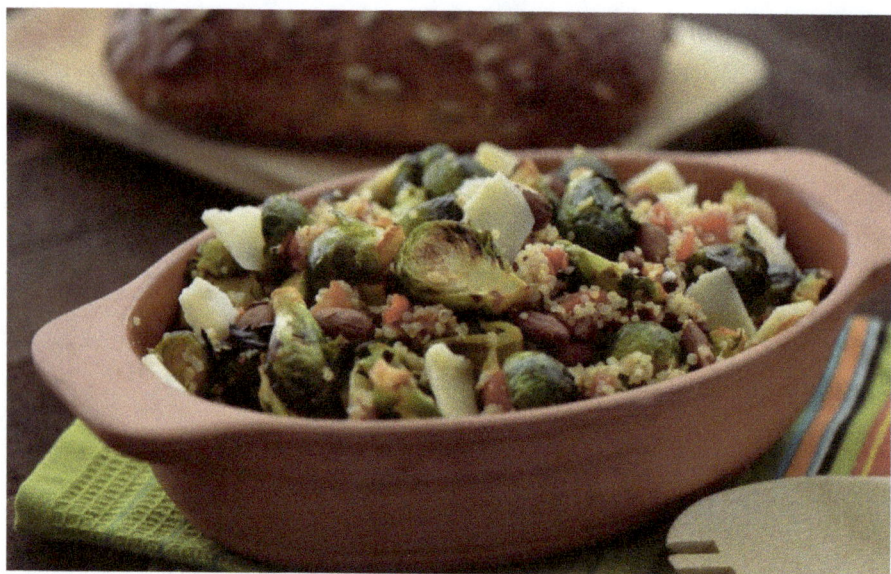

Pesto Tomato Cucumber Salad

Prep Time:
10 Minutes
Cook Time:
0 Minutes
Serve: 8

Ingredients:

- ½ cup Italian salad dressing
- ¼ cup prepared pesto
- 3 large tomatoes, sliced
- 2 medium cucumbers, halved and sliced
- 1 small red onion, sliced
- Salt and pepper to taste

Directions:

1. In a bowl, whisk the salad dressing and pesto.

2. Season with salt and pepper to taste.

3. Toss gently to incorporate everything.

4. Refrigerate before.

Nutrition: Calories: 82; Fat: 5g; Carbs: 7g; Protein: 2g

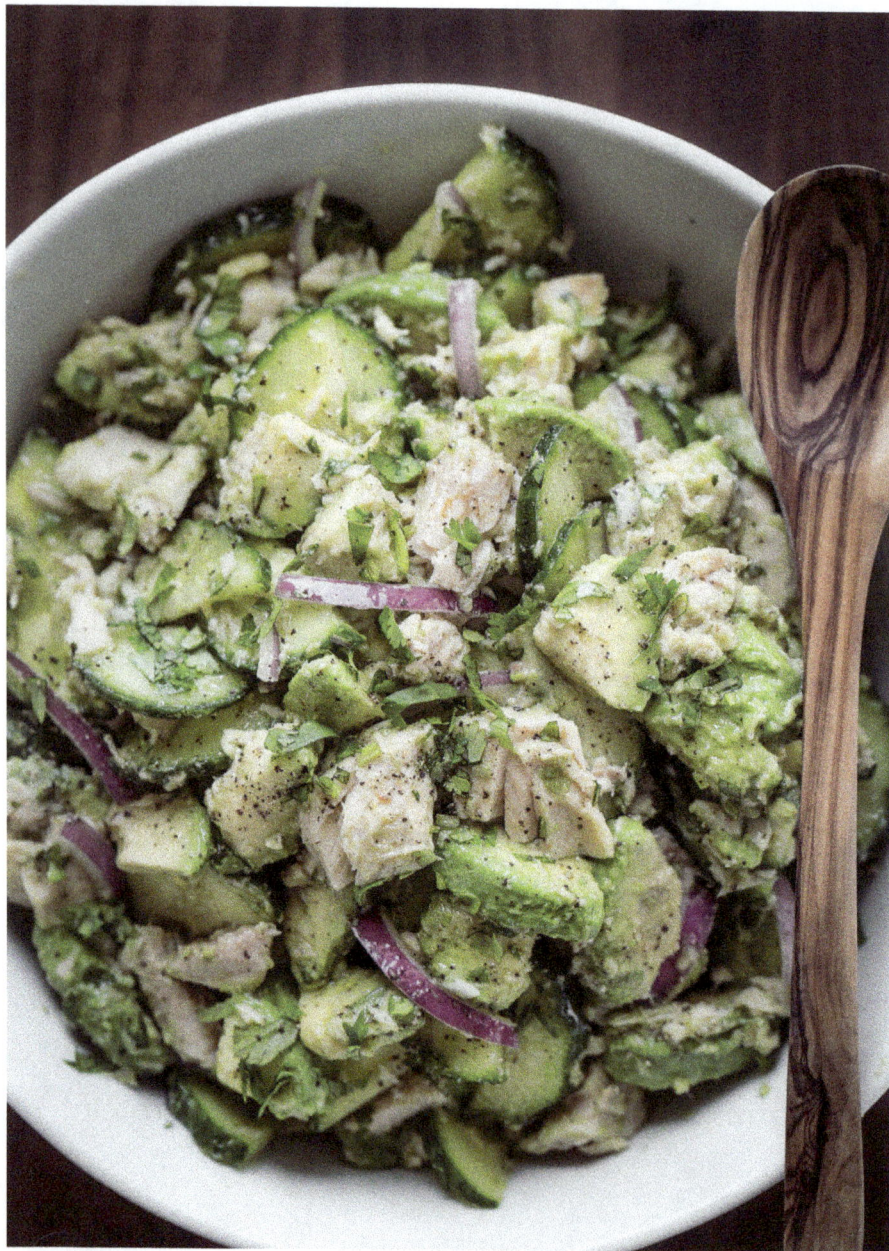

Easy Asian Style Chicken Slaw

Prep Time:
10 Minutes
Cook Time:
0 Minutes
Serve: 8

Ingredients:

- 3 ounces ramen noodles, cooked according to package
- 1 leftover rotisserie chicken, skin removed and shredded
- 16 ounces coleslaw mix
- 1 cup toasted sesame salad dressing
- 6 green onions, finely chopped
- Salt and pepper to taste

Directions:

1.Place the noodles in a bowl and top with the chicken and coleslaw mix.

2.Drizzle with sesame salad dressing and season with salt and pepper to taste.

3.Mix and garnish with green onions last.

Nutrition: Calories: 267; Fat: 10g; Carbs: 18g; Protein: 26g

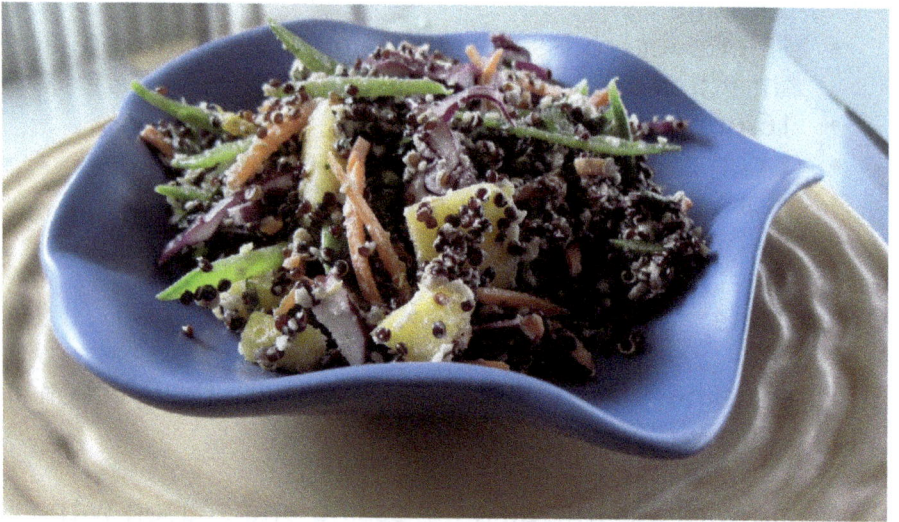

Cucumber and Red Onion Salad

Prep Time:
10 Minutes
Cook Time:
0 Minutes
Serve: 4

Ingredients:

- 2 small English cucumbers, sliced thinly
- 1 cup red onion, sliced thinly
- 2 tablespoons white wine vinegar
- ½ teaspoon sugar
- ¼ teaspoon sesame oil
- Salt and pepper to taste

Directions:

1.Put the cucumbers and red onions in a bowl.

2.In a small bowl, mix the white vinegar, sugar, and sesame oil. Season with salt and pepper to taste.

3.Pour over the cucumber and onions.

4.Toss to coat the ingredients.

Nutrition: Calories: 31; Fat: 1g; Carbs: 7g; Protein: 1g

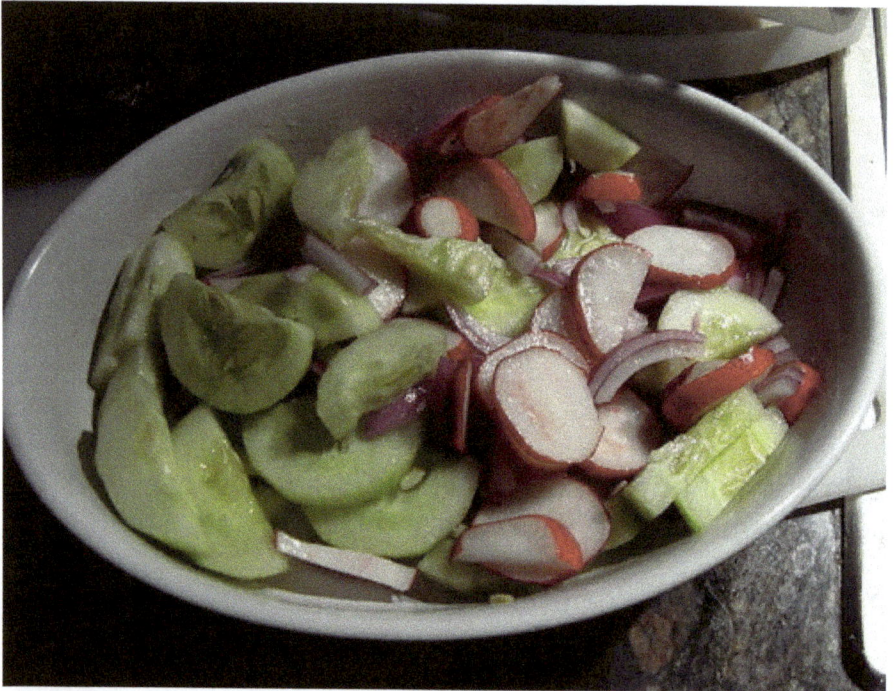

Bacon Tomato Salad

Prep Time:
15 Minutes
Cook Time:
0 Minutes
Serve: 6

Ingredients:

- 12 ounces iceberg lettuce blend
- 2 cups grape tomatoes, halved
- ¾ cup coleslaw salad dressing
- ¾ cup cheddar cheese, shredded
- 12 bacon strips, cooked and crumbled
- Salt and pepper to taste

Directions:

1.Put the lettuce and tomatoes in a salad bowl.

2.Drizzle with the dressing and sprinkle with cheese.

3.Season with salt and pepper to taste then mix.

4.Garnish with bacon bits on top.

Nutrition: Calories: 268; Fat: 20g; Carbs: 11g;
Protein: 10g

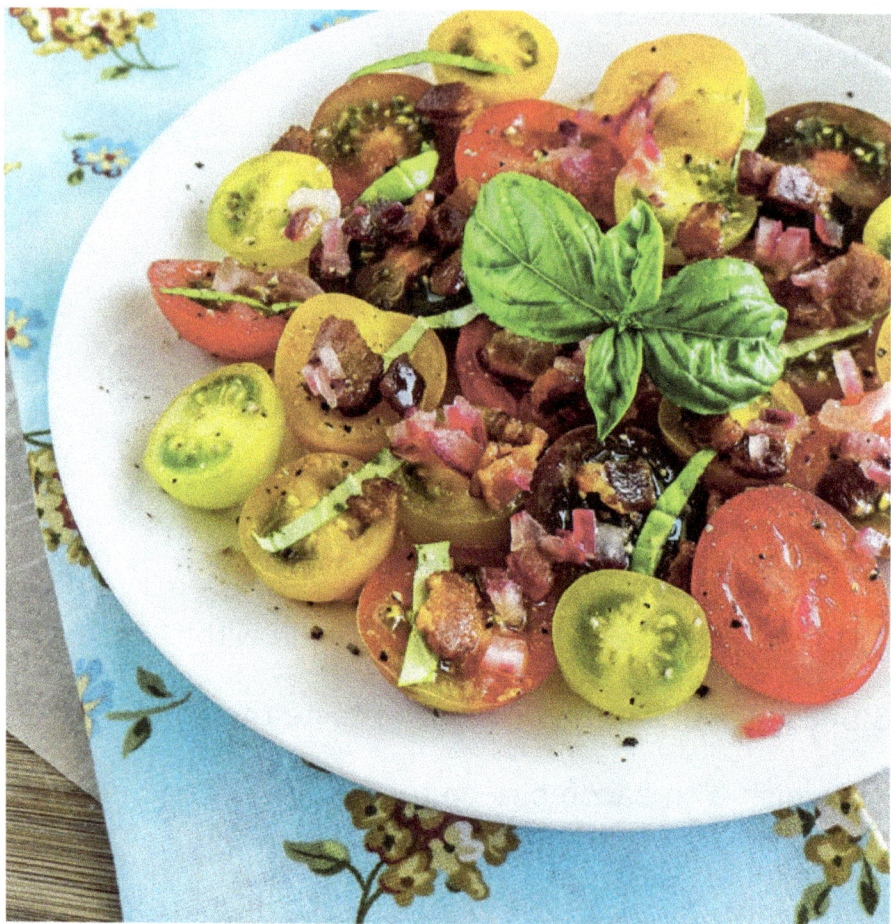

Easy Tea Cake

Prep Time:
10 minutes
Cook Time:
30 minutes
Serve: 12

Ingredients:

- 6 tablespoons green tea powder
- 2 cups almond milk
- 4 eggs
- 2 teaspoons vanilla extract
- 3 ½ cups almond flour
- 1 teaspoon baking soda
- 3 teaspoons baking powder

Directions:

1.In a bowl, mix the almond milk with green tea powder, eggs, vanilla, almond flour, baking soda and baking powder.

2.Stir until smooth then pour into a cake pan and place in the oven to bake at 350 degrees F for 30 minutes.

3.Slice and serve cold.

Nutrition: calories 170, fat 4, fiber 9, carbs 6, protein 5 581.

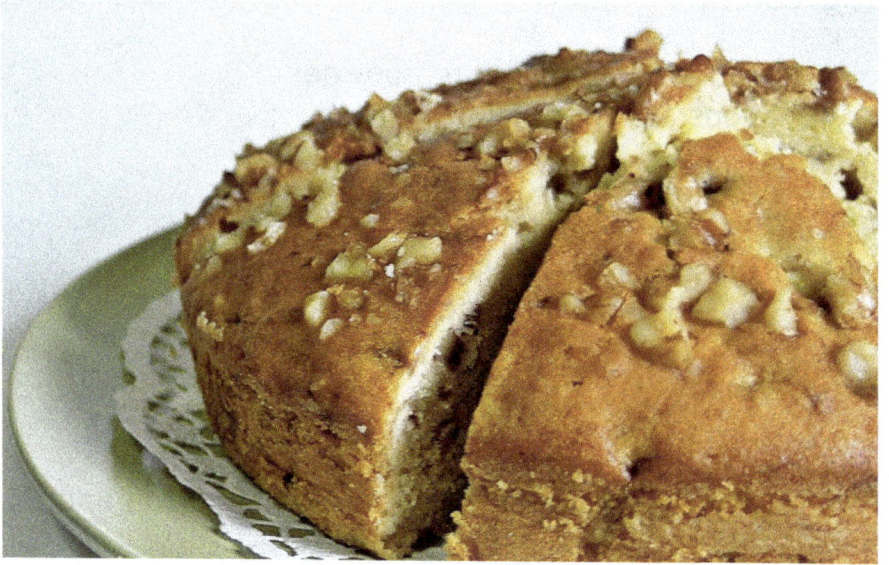

Coconut Cream

Prep Time:
2 hours
Cook Time:
5 minutes
Serve: 6

Ingredients:

- 14 ounces almond milk
- 14 ounces coconut cream
- 1 teaspoon gelatin powder

Directions:

1.In a pan, mix the almond milk with the cream and gelatin.

2.Stir, bring to a simmer over medium heat and cook for 5 minutes.

3. Divide into bowls and serve after 2 hours in the fridge.

Nutrition: calories 130, fat 4, fiber 3, carbs 7, protein 4 582.

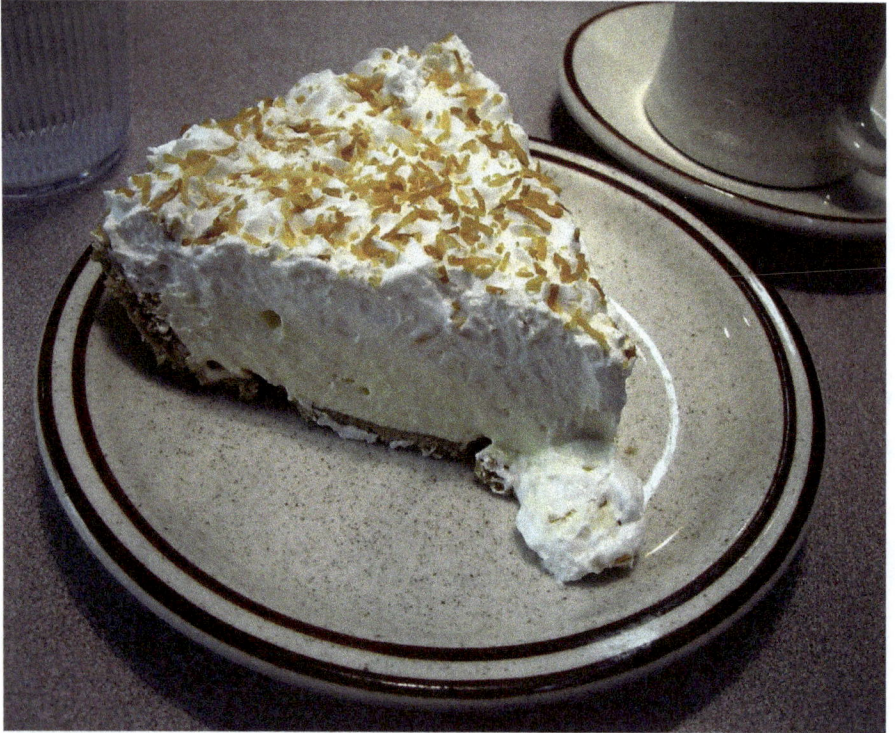

Creamy Cantaloupe Salad

Prep Time:
5 minutes
Cook Time:
0 minutes
Serve: 1

Ingredients:

- 1-ounce coconut cream
- 6 ounces cantaloupe, peeled and cubed
- A splash of lemon juice

Directions:

1.In a bowl, mix the cantaloupe with the cream and lemon juice.

2.Toss and serve.

Nutrition: calories 121, fat 6, fiber 2, carbs 15, protein 2 583.

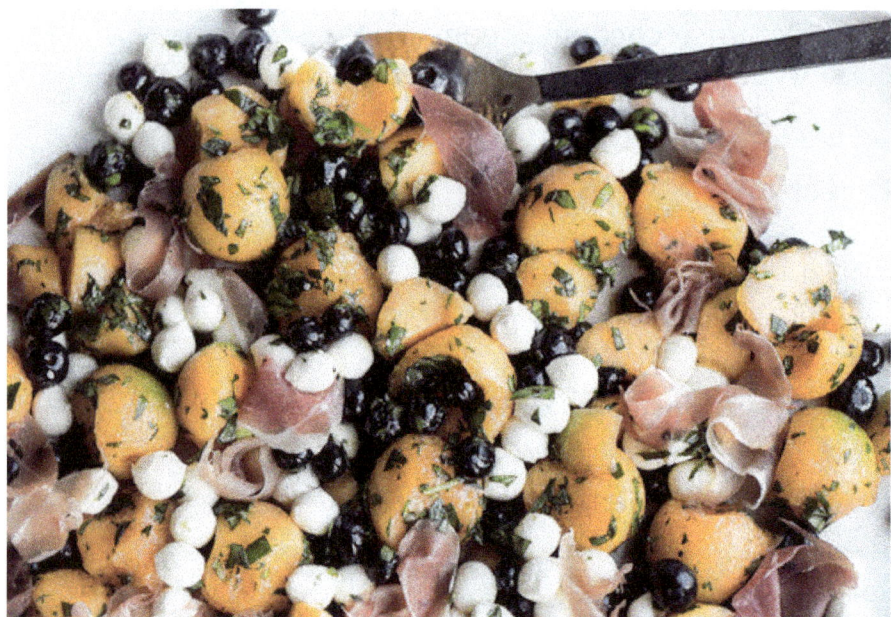